The
Road To
Wellness

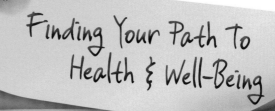

Finding Your Path To Health & Well-Being

Editorial Staff

Author: Dr. Brian Luke Seaward

Executive Editor: David Hunnicutt, PhD

Managing Editor: Brittanie Leffelman, MS

Contributing Editor: Carie Maguire

Creative Director: Brittany Stohl

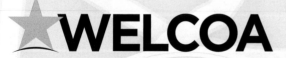

WELCOA

17002 Marcy Street, Suite 140 | Omaha, NE 68118
PH: 402-827-3590 | FX: 402-827-3594 | welcoa.org

Table of Contents

About WELCOA

The Wellness Council of America (WELCOA) was established as a national not-for-profit organization in the mid 1980s through the efforts of a number of forward-thinking business and health leaders. Drawing on the vision originally set forth by William Kizer, Sr., Chairman Emeritus of Central States Indemnity, and WELCOA founding Directors that included Dr. Louis Sullivan, former Secretary of Health and Human Services, and Warren Buffett, Chairman of Berkshire Hathaway, WELCOA has helped influence the face of workplace wellness in the U.S.

Today, WELCOA has become one of the most respected resources for workplace wellness in America. With a membership in excess of 5,000 organizations, WELCOA is dedicated to improving the health and well-being of all working Americans. Located in America's heartland, WELCOA makes its national headquarters in one of America's healthiest business communities—Omaha, Nebraska.

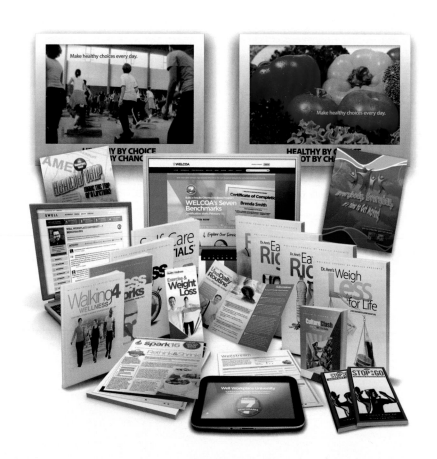

About **Brian Luke Seaward, PhD**

Brian Luke Seaward is a renowned and respected international expert in the fields of stress management, mind-body-spirit healing and corporate health promotion. Additionally, he is an award-winning author, photographer, teacher, celebrated film director/producer and much sought after inspirational speaker. His mission, as expressed through his legacy of acclaimed books and public appearances, is to make this a better world in which to live by having each of us reach our highest potential. Former Good Morning America host, Joan Lunden says, "Dr. Seaward's words have touched my life profoundly and helped me to find grace and dignity, the patience and compassion needed to navigate my ever-changing course. They have helped me understand that it is the way I choose to see the world that I will create the world I see." His corporate clients include Hewlett Packard, Procter & Gamble, Conoco Oil, Motorola, Quaker Oats, John Deere, BP-Amoco, Blue Cross/Blue Shield, Maxtor-Seagate, Organic Valley Dairy, US ARMY, and many others. He currently serves as the Executive Director of the Paramount Wellness Institute in Boulder, CO. Dr. Seaward can be reached via his website, **www.brianlukeseaward.net**.

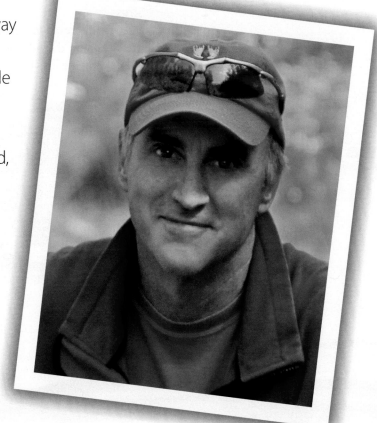

[FOREWORD]
From **Dr. Hunnicutt**

Although it's painful to say, we are on a crash course with a heartbreaking destiny—a tragic destiny that will affect tens of millions of Americans.

Indeed, unless important individual lifestyle changes are made, the typical American is about to lose their health status—and that is indeed, well, heartbreaking.

Consider the following:

Physical Activity
More than 60 percent of American adults do NOT get enough physical activity during the course of the day. In fact, 25% of U.S. adults do not get *any* physical activity at all.

Sadly, the consequences of not getting enough physical activity are legion. To be sure, not getting enough physical activity during the day increases the risk of dying prematurely from things like heart disease, cancer and diabetes. Moreover, a lack of physical activity means less energy, lower life satisfaction and a less optimistic outlook on the future.

Stress
More than three in four Americans regularly experience physical symptoms caused by stress—almost the same number routinely experience psychological manifestations caused by living lives that are out of balance.

From upset stomachs to headaches to sleepless nights, stress has become a major health problem—and endemic to our society.

Nutrition
According to the Centers for Disease Control and Prevention, more than two-thirds of Americans are carrying far too much weight. Tragically, the heartbreaking consequence of this reality is the fact that millions of people will experience major health concerns like type 2 diabetes, heart disease and cancer.

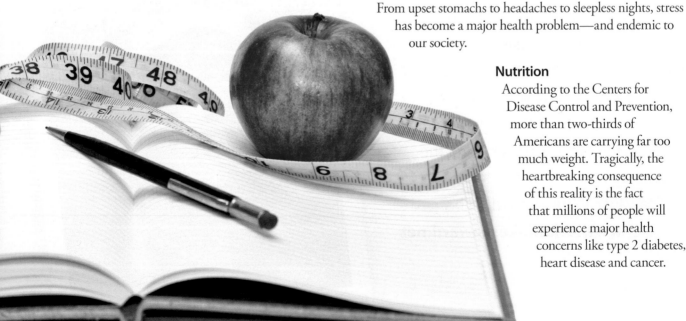

But even more concerning than just the physical manifestations of poor health practices is the notion that most people are leading lives that are woefully out of balance and dramatically out of sync.

It's easy to see that it's time for a change.

And that's where Dr. Brian Luke Seaward enters the picture.

I've known Dr. Seaward for more than 20 years and, like millions of others, have followed his work with great interest. To my delight, when I discovered his availability I made it a point to lock him into this project.

In his book, *The Road To Wellness*, Dr. Seaward takes you down the path of personal discovery. With honesty, accuracy and compassion, he'll share with you what it will take for you to experience your best you—and if you follow his advice, you can indeed lead a life of meaning, vitality and purpose.

The formula for the book is a simple one.

There are seven chapters. Each addresses a different component of well-being. Importantly, each chapter is filled with useful information—information that can make your life better. At the end of each chapter, there are personal opportunities for self-reflections and goal setting.

By working through the material thoughtfully and methodically you will not only understand what will be required for you to make the changes that are necessary for you to lead a whole and fulfilled life, but you will actually see the changes start to materialize.

As you begin your journey on *The Road To Wellness*, I encourage you to embrace the opportunity to see the world in a new light and to do things differently. Amazingly, small tweaks in your daily life will lead to amazing outcomes.

From where I sit, there is no question that this book is the first step on the road to a life well-lived.

Enjoy your journey!

Yours in good health,

David Hunnicutt, PhD
CEO
Wellness Council of America

About
Dr. David Hunnicutt

Since his arrival at WELCOA in 1995, David Hunnicutt, PhD has developed countless publications that have been widely adopted in businesses and organizations throughout North America. Known for his ability to make complex issues easier to understand, David has a proven track-record of publishing health and wellness material that helps employees lead healthier lifestyles. David travels extensively advocating better health practices and radically different thinking in organizations of all kinds.

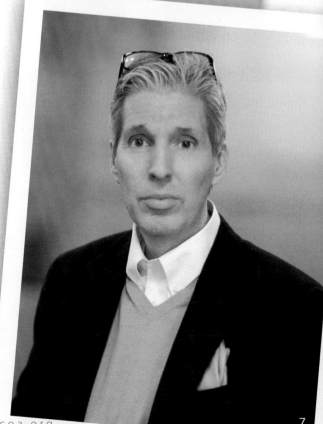

[CHAPTER 1]

The Good Life... Revisited

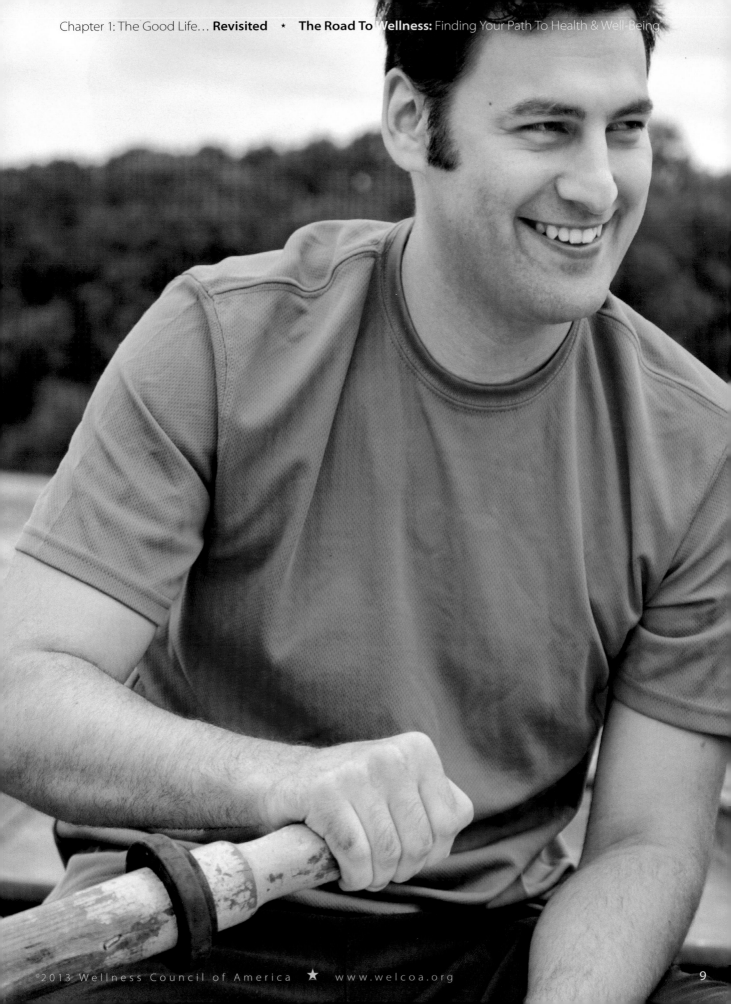

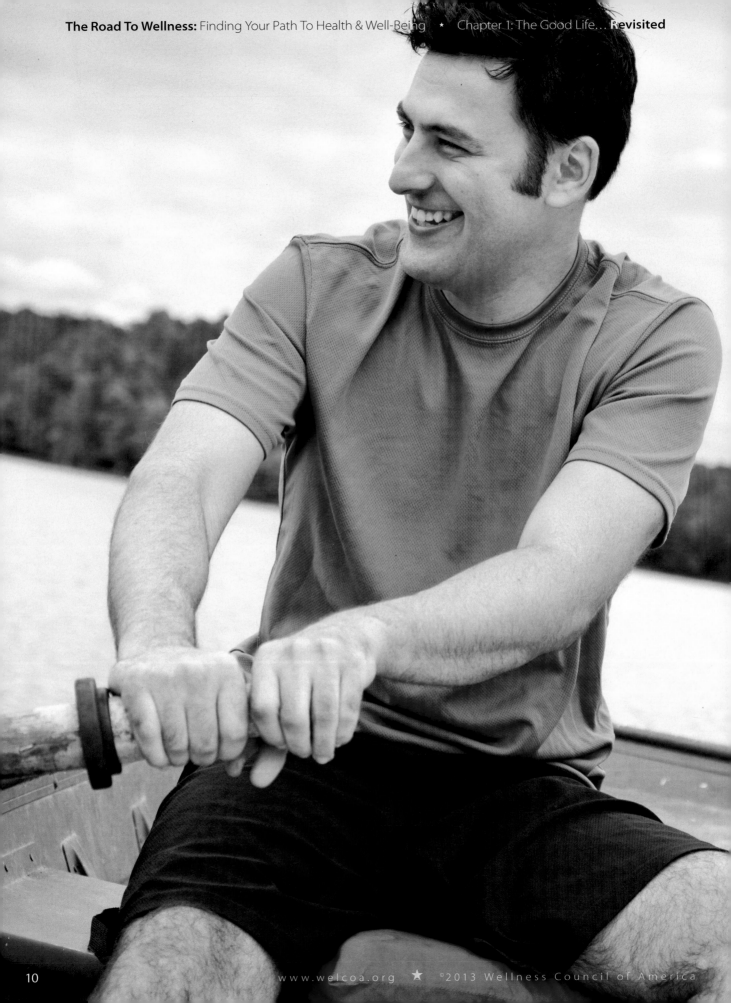

[CHAPTER 1]

The Good Life... Revisited

Anne gets up every morning around sunrise and heads to a nature preserve called Golden Ponds. With her camera in hand, she walks the four mile loop briskly before hopping back in the car and heading off to work. I see Anne every morning as I walk my dog. Occasionally, she shares some of her photos, like the day she proudly showed me the image of the two red fox cubs on the prowl, the river minx, the bald eagle snacking on a trout or the small herd of mule deer staring down a coyote. With each photo her eyes light up like a child, and she smiles ear to ear. Anne confided in me that she has lost 30 pounds walking every morning, but that's not why she walks. "I come out early to commune with nature," she says. "It's a great way to put perspective in your life." Anne always ends her conversations the same way. "Life is good!" she says, with another smile. Indeed it is.

Welcome to the good life! What exactly does "the good life" mean today? To a teenager, the good life means freedom, usually expressed as a new video game, or a car with a full tank of gas. To a corporate executive or factory worker, the good life means a decent paycheck and quality time spent with one's children. To a newly retired senior, the good life might mean traveling abroad, or a regular golf tee time. To an octogenarian, the good life might translate to a day without physical pain. The good life is something we all strive for, yet it's neither a fantasy, nor a reward. The good life is a

"Life is good!"

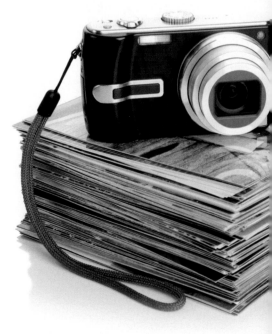

mindset for health and happiness. And while some may see it as a birthright, the truth is no matter who we are or how old we may be, the good life is as much a responsibility as a gift. First and foremost the good life is an uncompromising attitude to live a responsible, well-balanced life. Let there be no doubt, in a world filled with stressors, distractions and challenges, this attitude will be tested often, yet never vanquished. In the wise words of renowned psychologist, Carl Rogers, "The good life is a process, not a state of being. It is a direction, not a destination." British philosopher, Bertrand Russell, said it like this: "The good life is one inspired by love and guided by knowledge."

The good life doesn't just happen; it takes dedication, inspiration and at times, a fair bit of perspiration. Anyone who has walked a proverbial mile in this direction will tell you it is certainly worth it. Perhaps the expression "the good life" can be summed up easily in this phrase: A sense of inner peace. Those people who have lived long enough to share their wisdom are quick to point out that a new car, a beautiful house or a healthy stock portfolio are meaningless if one's health is compromised. These same people remind us repeatedly of this sage advice: When you have your health, you have everything. So, the mindset of the good life begins with optimal wellness.

The Roots Of Wellness

The word "wellness" is relatively new to the American vernacular, but the concept of wellness is ageless. The term wellness is based on the timeless concept of wholeness, where the whole is always greater than the sum of its parts. The universal symbol of wholeness is a circle. Think of the sun, the full moon or even our planet and you get the idea. So powerful is the symbol of the circle as a message of wholeness that it is used countless ways in our culture—dinner plates, clocks, Christmas wreaths, coins, wedding bands and the peace symbol are just a few of the countless examples. Many companies even use the symbol of the circle in their corporate logos.

If you were to talk to the shamans, sages, healers and wisdom keepers of all cultures and ages and ask them "What are the parts that make up the whole regarding wellness?" you would hear them answer with four aspects: mind, body, spirit and emotions. They might even draw a circle then divide it into four equal parts labeling each one, mental well-being, physical well-being, emotional well-being and spiritual well-being, respectively. Of course, these lines really don't exist because there is no separation between mind and body or spirit and emotions. It is all one incredible dynamic package. We merely draw these lines to help understand each wellness quadrant better (much like this book). The essence of "the good life" is living the "whole" picture.

> "The good life is a process, not a state of being. It is a direction, not a destination."
> – Carl Rogers

What is the best definition of wellness? Let's start with this: Wellness is the integration, balance and harmony of mind, body, spirit and emotions where the whole is always greater than the sum of the parts for optimal health.

In the Western culture the focus on wellness tends to place the greatest importance on physical health (mainly because this is the easiest to measure—think bone density, cholesterol and blood pressure). Yet, by ignoring one or more of the other components we do a great injustice to our overall well-being. Simply stated, we compromise our quality of life. The "good life" not only honors, but engages in the ageless concept of wellness: the integration, balance and harmony of mind, body spirit and emotions where the whole is always greater than the sum of the parts. Here is a closer look at each aspect:

Physical Well-Being: The optimal functioning of all the body's physiological systems (e.g., the immune system, the cardiovascular system, the neuromuscular system, etc.)

With repeated headline news about coronary heart disease, strokes, diabetes and obesity, most wellness programs place their focus here with an emphasis on aerobic exercise and some muscular strength. Physical well-being also includes healthy nutrition, quality sleep and the art of relaxation to reduce the symptoms of stress.

Emotional Well-Being: The ability to feel and express the entire range of human emotions (from anger to love, but the point is to control these emotions, not be controlled by them). The spectrum of human emotions is quite large; yet some aspects are lauded and others are considered taboo (anger and fear). Today, there is great interest in the pursuit of happiness but emotional well-being covers them all, from healthy grieving and creative anger management to joy, happiness and comic relief.

Mental Well-Being: The ability to gather, process, recall and communicate information. Much like a computer, our mind, comprised of intellect, intuition and imagination, is nothing less than amazing, yet these cognitive skills for information processing need to be cultivated on a regular basis. However, when the mind gets overwhelmed with sensory bombardment, (think smart phones, Facebook, iPads, text messaging, Twitter, emails, YouTube, Pinterest, etc.) the ability to gather, process, recall and communicate information is greatly compromised. Mental well-being includes, but is not limited to tools to calm the mind (meditation) as well as sharpening it (creative problem solving).

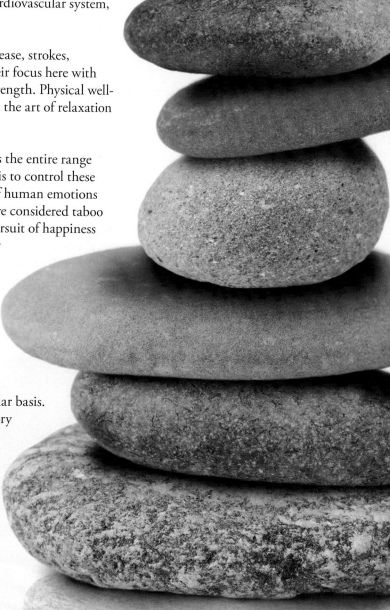

> The "good life" not only honors, but engages in the ageless concept of wellness...

> " If we don't honor the integration, balance and harmony of mind, body, spirit and emotions, we are going to end up with a dysfunctional life."

Spiritual Well-Being: This often neglected component involves the elevation of consciousness as it relates to three aspects of the human condition: relationships, values and a meaningful purpose in life. Not the same thing as religion, (though they share common ground) human spirituality involves nurturing your conscience in times of stress through the inner resources of patience, forgiveness, compassion, optimism, faith, integrity and many, many more. Wisdom keepers remind us that a meaningful purpose in life is the cornerstone of spiritual well-being. Research shows that a lack of a meaningful purpose in life can greatly compromise one's physical well-being.

So common are these four aspects of wellness that various terms like "mental health day," "emotional intelligence," "emotional literacy," "a spiritual experience," and "health of the human spirit," are often heard in everyday conversations, and are now even tweeted and posted on Facebook updates. So when you think about health and wellness, realize this covers more than just aerobics and broccoli! As the saying goes, "If we don't honor the integration, balance and harmony of mind, body, spirit and emotions, we are going to end up with a dysfunctional life."

Dysfunction: A Good Life Threatened?

Many health and wellness issues we face today were simply unheard of in our grandparent's time. In fact, many of these issues were unheard of in our parent's time. While it's true that every age has had its challenges to live a healthy lifestyle, from the Black Plague to epidemics of polio and tuberculosis, the dawn of the 21st century is no exception. To update Charles Dickens' most famous opening line, "It's the best of times (a great standard of living) and the worst of times" (financial chaos, climate change and global terrorism). As a whole, Americans we have it quite good, but we also have some serious problems to deal with, both individually and collectively. There is no time like the present to start. Moreover, people who keep their fingers on the pulse of society warn of potential health crises on the horizon including, but not limited to the following: lack of exposure to natural sunlight, (vitamin D deficiency) techno-stress and Internet addictions, a rise of cancer, heart disease, diabetes and Alzheimer's disease and repeated exposure to toxic chemicals in the environment. Despite these challenges, we are not powerless. Quite the contrary and this message underscores the importance of striving to live the good life.

21ST CENTURY WELLNESS STATISTICS

> The typical person spends 95 percent of his/her day indoors.

> As many as one-third of Americans are prescribed anti-depressants.

> Over 50 percent of Americans claim to get a poor night's sleep.

> The typical American eats one or more meals outside of their home.

> The average person consumes their body weight in refined sugar each year.

> On average, people receive 50 to 100 emails a day and countless text messages.

> An ever-increasing number of Americans are considered either overweight or obese.

There is a concept in wellness circles called wellness robbers, which are the things that steal our ability to live a healthy lifestyle. Unlike thugs, crooks and burglars, these wellness robbers fall in two categories: things we can control and things we cannot. Wellness experts remind us repeatedly to start with the wellness robbers we can control, including those behaviors in which we rob from ourselves (e.g., poor eating habits, excessive time with screen technology, poor sleep hygiene, etc.) How is your overall health status? What aspects of health in your life do you feel are stolen from you? Exercise 1.1 and 1.2 invite you to take a closer look.

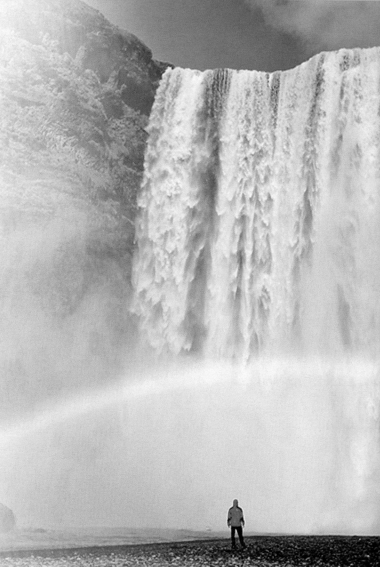

From Good To Great:
The Winds Of Change

Sometimes it takes a crisis to put important aspects of your life into focus. Such was the case of Janice. At the age of 34, Janice felt like she was on top of the world; a great career, a solid marriage, a beautiful home and an adorable five year old daughter. Sure, there were many long days at the office (it's to be expected, she would say) and perhaps one too many cups of coffee (truth be told, she lived on caffeine) and vacation resorts had to be places with WiFi (no national parks). Despite all of this, Janice felt like she was at the pinnacle of success. Her friends and colleagues thought so too. So did her husband (who earned much less than she did). Life was good, but in hindsight, Janice would say this was an illusion. Things were definitely not in balance.

The winds of change can rise suddenly and swiftly. It was these same winds that knocked Janice off balance in a matter of seconds. It happened like this: One morning during her annual checkup, her physician revealed that she had ovarian cancer. The first stage of grieving is shock, quickly followed by denial. Then comes anger. Janice experienced all three at once. Her first words were, "Cancer? I don't have time for cancer in my life." It was those same words that

> *Even if you're on the right track, you'll get run over if you just sit there.*
>
> —Will Rogers

gave her pause for thought. After a good cathartic cry and a hug from her husband, Janice made a promise to herself. She was going to create new priorities in her life, starting with a better balance between work and her life at home. "I was living a life without a foundation," she explained. Today, five years later Janice is cancer free and quite happy, but this new lifestyle didn't happen overnight. "I sat down and examined my life and made some significant changes. It's funny how a curveball like cancer can really make you reprioritize your life. Despite the initial shock, this disease is the best thing that has ever happened to me," she said. "I made a plan to get back on my feet and live again—to be the victor, not the victim. My husband calls it a blueprint. Regardless of what you call it, this strategy not only saved my life, it became my life and I am forever grateful."

Creating A Wellness Blueprint: Goal Setting

Before you set off on a trip, it's best to pack the right clothes and have some sense of where you're going. Living the good life is much the same way. To live a healthy, well-balanced life, you need to have a solid game plan, and before you start planning the details, it's best to make a list of goals. In the words of Will Rogers, "Even if you're on the right track, you'll get run over if you just sit there." Speaking of goals, if you ever get a chance, make a point to see the documentary *Into the Void*, which is a remarkable story about two mountain climbers. One climber, left for dead, returns back to civilization with a broken leg by making hundreds of small, but persistent goals to survive and make it back down the mountain.

People have been studying and analyzing the concept of goal setting for eons and this much we know for sure:

1. Be specific about what you want. Over-riding goals are great (e.g., "I am healthy") but specifics (e.g., "I snack on fruits and nuts") are essential too!

2. Effective changes don't happen over night, they take time (so be patient). Although you may see and feel some results early on, decades of research reveal that it takes about six to eight weeks to see any significant changes. So be patient. Long-term goals are great, but take it one day at a time.

3. Make a habit to state and repeat your goal every day. Repeating your goals out loud will have a positive influence on your behaviors.

4. Goals should be stated in the present tense and be positive (e.g., I go to bed at 10:00 p.m. every night). Remember, your unconscious mind governs your behavior and the unconscious mind's first preference of thought is the affirmative. Negative thoughts like "I don't want to gain 10 more pounds" are interpreted as "I want to gain 10 more pounds." Olympic athletes will tell you that it helps to put a mental image with the goal (the unconscious mind loves images and symbols).

5. Roadblocks and distractions are part of the journey. Everyone has setbacks. Rosa Parks, Michael Phelps, Nelson Mandala and Robert Redford all had setbacks. Setbacks (even slip-ups) are said to be part of the learning process. And remember it's OK to stop and smell the roses too (just don't derail your life with pit-stops). Guilt trips, while not uncommon, can become an unnecessary detour to your destination. So acknowledge the moment, then get back on track.

Worksheet Exercise 1.3 will help you get started on your personal wellness goals.

Are you ready to live (or continue living) a good life? Great! Like Exercise 1.3, this book has many concepts and additional worksheet exercises to help you create (or perhaps fine tune) your path to wellness. While there is no specific recipe for optimal wellness that is right for everyone, this we do know: Will power, determination, moderation and a good sense of humor will help to guide you along the way. Please use the information and exercises in this book as your roadmap and compass to help you chart your best path to wellness and the good life. Remember, there is no one way to create the essence of a good life; there are many ways.

> "Remember, there is no one way to create the essence of a good life; there are many ways."

[EXERCISE 1.1]

My Picture Of Health & Wellness

We all have an idea of what ideal health is. Many of us take our health for granted until something goes wrong to remind us that our picture of health is compromised and less than ideal. Although health may seem to be objective, it will certainly vary from person to person over the entire aging process. The following statements are based on characteristics associated with longevity and a healthy quality of life (none of which considers any genetic factors). Rather than answering the basic question "how long will I live?" please complete this inventory to determine your current picture of health.

	3 = Often	2 = Sometimes	1 = Rarely	0 = Never
1. With rare exception, I sleep on average 7 to 8 hours each night.	3	2	1	0
2. I tend to eat my meals at the same time each day.	3	2	1	0
3. I keep my bedtime consistent every night.	3	2	1	0
4. I do cardiovascular exercise at least three times per week.	3	2	1	0
5. My weight is considered ideal for my height.	3	2	1	0
6. Without exception, my alcohol consumption is in moderation.	3	2	1	0
7. I consider my nutritional habits to be exceptional.	3	2	1	0
8. My health status is considered excellent, with no pre-existing conditions.	3	2	1	0
9. I neither smoke, nore participate in the use of recreational drugs.	3	2	1	0
10. I have a solid group of friends with whom I socialize regularly.	3	2	1	0
TOTAL SCORE ❯				

SCORE

26-30 points = Excellent health habits   14-19 points = Questionable health habits

20-25 points = Moderate health habits   0-13 points = Poor health habits

[EXERCISE 1.2]

Do You Have Wellness Robbers Lurking Around?

Who or what steals from your good life bounty? By discovering the things that rob us of our highest wellness potential we can begin to makes changes to regain our inner balance and personal fortitude. Take a few minutes to identify any and all robbers by listing them here in each of the four wellness categories. Please keep in mind that some wellness robbers may show up in more than one wellness component.

Physical Well-Being

1. _____
2. _____
3. _____
4. _____
5. _____

Emotional Well-Being

1. _____
2. _____
3. _____
4. _____
5. _____

Mental Well-Being

1. _____
2. _____
3. _____
4. _____
5. _____

Spiritual Well-Being

1. _____
2. _____
3. _____
4. _____
5. _____

Please write any additional thoughts, insights, and comments on this topic here:

[EXERCISE 1.3]

My Personal Wellness Goals

Most people begin behavioral changes with a simple goal; to be healthy. What over-riding wellness goal do you wish to manifest in your life at this time? Sometimes, by actually writing down our thoughts, goals, wishes and dreams, this specific action becomes the first step in making it really happen. Putting pen to paper becomes an unofficial contract we make with ourselves for self-improvement or simply a step toward personal happiness. Please take a moment to write down an over-riding goal you have about your health and well-being here:

My overall wellness goal is: _____

_____

An over-riding goal, like a foundation to a house is a good start, but you cannot live on a foundation—more structure is required. Simply stated, more detail is needed to make this dream come to fruition. Specifics are essential. Using the architecture metaphor, we need walls, a roof, insulation, dry wall, plumbing and electricity. With this in mind, what are some specifics to add to your foundation that will make your over-riding wellness goals actually happen?

Specific Health & Wellness Goals:

1. _____
2. _____
3. _____
4. _____
5. _____

Additional Goals:

6. _____
7. _____
8. _____
9. _____
10. _____

In this day and age, it is so easy to become distracted (even disenchanted) with our life plans. Staying focused and motivated is essential. For this reason, once you have completed this worksheet, consider posting a copy on your refrigerator or bathroom mirror to remind you to maintain a focus of these goals. Finally, here are some words to consider about goal setting from motivational expert, Denis Waitley:

> " Learn from the past, set vivid details and goals for the future, and live in the only moment of which you have control—now. "

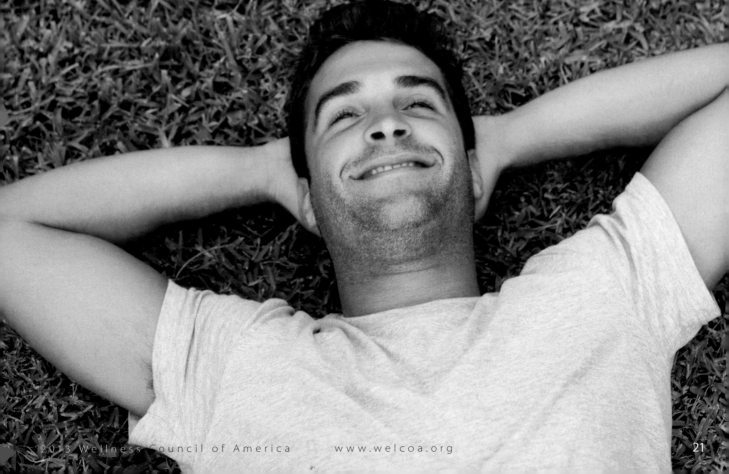

"You are never too old to set another goal or dream a new dream."

– C.S. Lewis

[CHAPTER 2]

Creating Healthy Boundaries

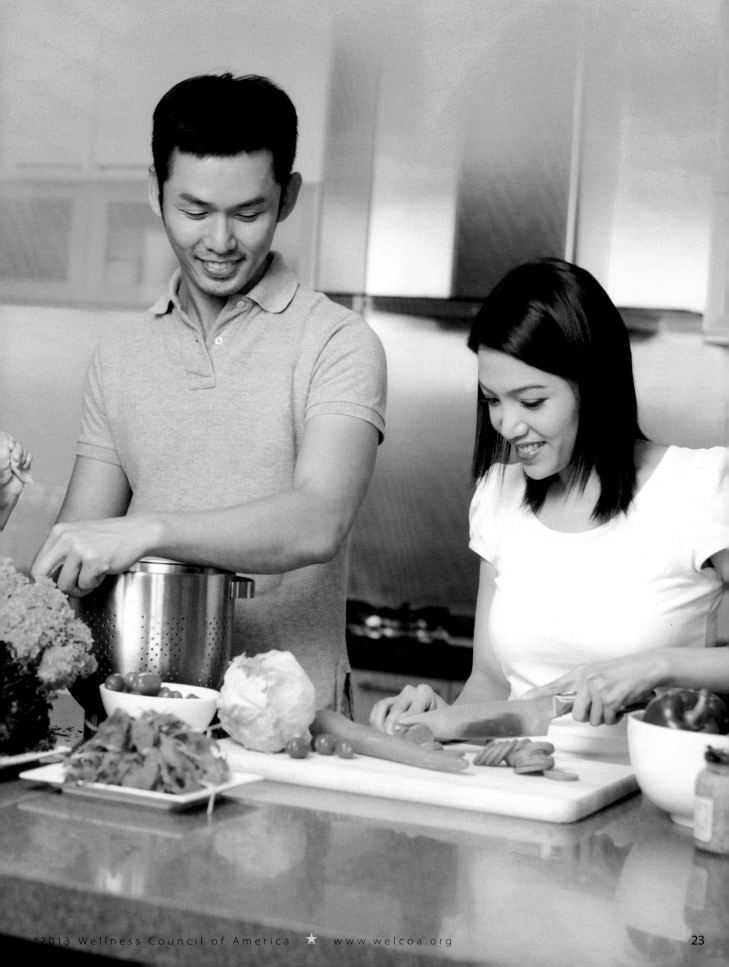

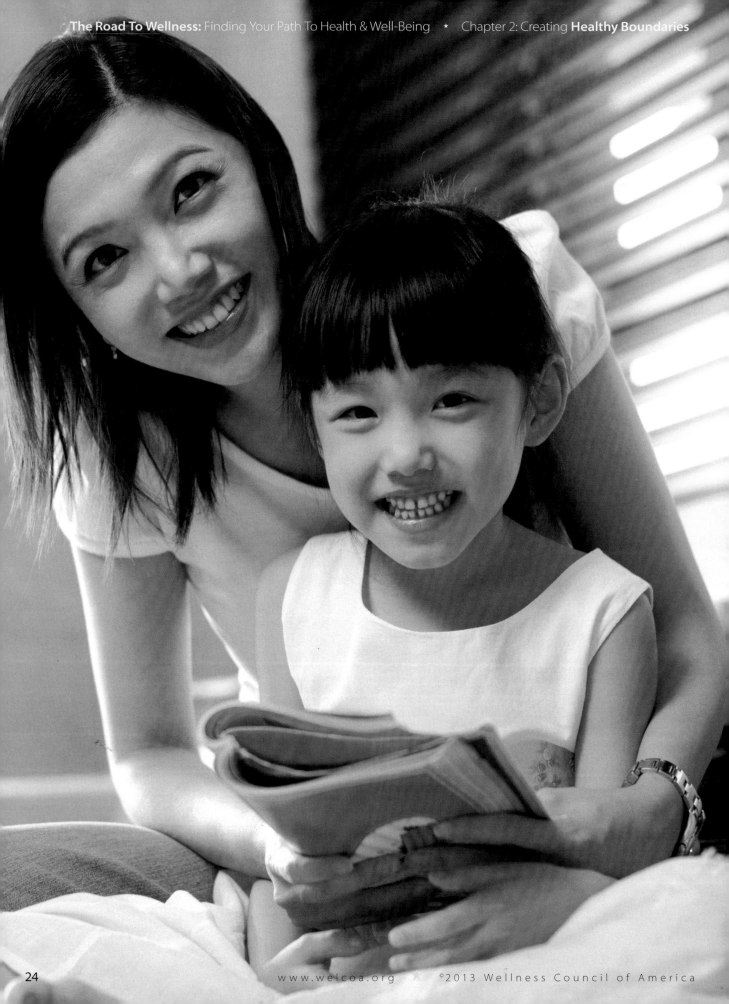

[CHAPTER 2]

Creating Healthy Boundaries

L ike most people today, Lynn has a smart phone. Unlike most people, Lynn has adopted a strong set of healthy boundaries with its use. "Technology is supposed to be a servant to us, yet ironically, I see so many people today becoming slaves to technology, especially with their cell phones. Not me. Life is too short to be a slave. I turn my cell phone off unless I intend to make a call. We lived for eons without cell phones, but you would never know it in this day and age. If I don't answer my phone, please leave a message… or call back. It's that simple," she says without any hint of sarcasm.

If you have ever been a parent, (and even if you have not) you have heard of the developmental stage of childhood called "The Terrible Twos." It's the age when infants, upon finding their voice, use the word "NO!" with great, perhaps incessant freedom. It's at this moment in time when parents begin to lay down the law. Indeed, we first learn about healthy boundaries from our parents: *Eat your vegetables. Do your homework. Brush your teeth. Be in bed by 8:30 p.m.* It's every child's job to push these boundaries, and it's every parent's job to hold firm. Boundaries, however, are not just for kids. They are for everyone!

Healthy boundaries provide structure, and quite often, stability in our lives. Consider one of the smallest parts of your body, the cell. All cells, from muscle tissue to blood cells, have cell membranes. Like a city wall that protects the

> 66 Healthy boundaries provide structure, and quite often, stability in our lives. 99

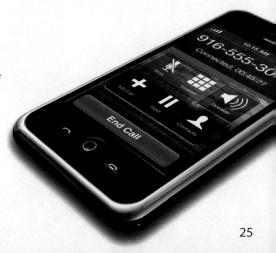

The good news is that establishing new boundaries for health and optimal wellness can begin today.

mighty castle and cozy hamlet inside, boundaries offer protection and stability. Cell membranes regulate what comes in and what goes out. Without cell membranes, complete havoc would ensue and ultimately destroy the cell's integrity. Rivers have banks for much the same reason. When river waters exceed their banks, all hell breaks loose. The same can be said for our lives: Without healthy boundaries to guide our daily behaviors, all hell breaks loose, whether it's addictions, chronic disease, compromising relationships, financial distress or all of these things together (YIKES!). Could the reins of your life be pulled in a little? If so, you are not alone. In fact, you are in excellent company. Poor health boundaries are rampant in American culture. Poor health boundaries not only erode the foundation for a good life, they can shake the ground the foundation rests upon like a high magnitude earth quake. The good news is that establishing new boundaries for health and optimal wellness can begin today. Everyone needs healthy boundaries, and these boundaries need constant attention. Exercise 2.1, *Creating Healthy Boundaries*, invites you to examine your life through the lens of healthy boundaries, and where necessary, make a new attempt at regaining a foothold of personal stability in your life.

Literally and figuratively speaking, healthy boundaries (also called healthy habits) provide a sense of responsibility; they not only provide balance to the inherent desire for freedom, but they also provide a great measure of integrity to your life as well. Freedom without responsibility is dangerous; ultimately it can be quite hazardous. So it is with all aspects of life: Freedom must be balanced with responsibility. Those who have been to college can attest to this struggle between freedom and responsibility. Regardless of when you leave the proverbial nest to fly off on your own, this process of establishing healthy boundaries may take years, if not decades to perfect as you navigate the course of your life. Indeed, children are given boundaries by their parents, grandparents and even teachers. However, once you mature into adulthood, you become responsible to establish your own set of healthy boundaries. We all know how this story goes. We establish rules to live by, (from those New Year's resolutions to fad diets to 12-step programs) yet they are all too easily ignored, and then forgotten. No doubt, pulling the reins in our lives is no small task! The good news is that it's not impossible either. It takes determination and commitment. Simply stated: Healthy boundaries are the cornerstone to the good life.

The term "healthy boundaries" can be distilled down to this simple message: Appropriate behavior; *Cover your mouth when you sneeze, don't use your cell phone at the cinema, or drive only when sober.* Some healthy boundaries are imposed upon us. Take for example people who become allergic to wheat products and then can only eat "gluten free" foods. Most healthy boundaries, however, are less dogmatic, yet equally important, for they become necessary steps in which to live a life of optimal wellness. Moreover, healthy boundaries offer a means for resiliency when we meet the unexpected. Indeed, healthy boundaries become the behaviors we invest in to ensure a healthy life.

It's fair to say that most of our major health issues today result from poor health boundaries. Lack of exercise, poor nutritional habits, sloppy sleep habits, unwise financial habits; the list is nearly endless… and the results can be nothing less than catastrophic. Technology in the information age has added a whole new spin to poor health boundaries. Exercise 2.2, *Master or Slave?* is a survey that offers a look at the newest health issue: Screen addictions.

We have all heard the expression, "Too much of a good thing is bad." Ageless wisdom reminds us (repeatedly) that moderation is key to a good life. Hence, one of the keys to the good life is establishing and practicing the art of healthy boundaries. Simply stated: Healthy boundaries provide a means to pull the reins in on our lives and gain a sense of balance also known as empowerment. Sage advice reminds us to do so before irreparable harm is done to the mind, body or spirit. Boundaries can be both confining and liberating. It all depends on your attitude, which ironically is also considered a healthy boundary.

> " Hence, one of the keys to the good life is establishing and practicing the art of healthy boundaries. "

Whining: The First Sign Of Poor Boundaries?

Jenny is a whiner. She whines about everything, from the traffic driving to work and the rising cost of groceries to photocopier jams and relentless evening telemarketers. To hear Jenny whine would make you think that she has a lot of stress in her life (most of which she creates herself) and that her life is horrible. By all accounts, Jenny, like most Americans, has it extremely good, yet you would never know it listening to her complain about how bad things are. Jenny is not alone in this common, but less than desirable behavior. Experts in the field of sociology suggest that ironically, in a nation of abundance, whining has become a national pastime. In psychology circles, whining is known as "victimization" where the person complaining wears the invisible, but recognizable label of "victim" on their forehead. Simply stated, whining is a form of grieving—grieving the loss of an expectation. And while grieving is considered healthy, even this behavior needs healthy boundaries. Prolonged grieving in the form of whining gets old fast. As the expression goes, "Once a victim, twice a volunteer."

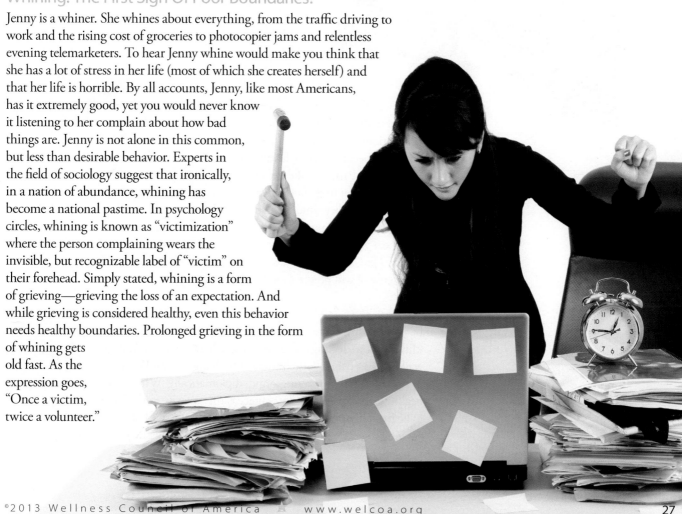

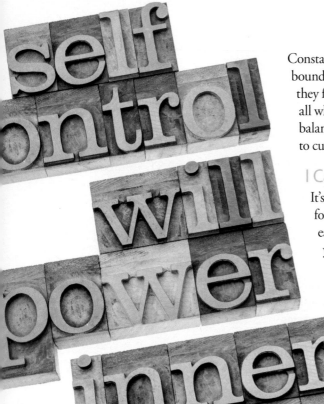

self control will power inner peace

Constant whining is not only a sign of grieving, it is also a sign of poor health boundaries—in this case emotional boundaries. Indeed, people grieve when they feel violated, and justifiably so. Having healthy boundaries won't stop all whining, but undoubtedly, they will empower you to feel a better sense of balance in your life. Exercise 2.3, *Cheese With Your Whine?* offers a new habit to curb an old pastime. Please give it a try.

I Can… And I Will: Creating Healthy Habits

It's not enough just to have healthy boundaries. These personal guidelines for healthy living have to be honored by putting them into practice—each and every day. Like leaning to play an instrument or perfecting your golf swing, every behavior takes practice, and lots of it until it becomes second nature. This means that the first few attempts may not look successful. In fact, you may fail miserably, and that's OK! No one ever said changing behaviors was easy. Practice and more practice is the key until it becomes a routine, woven seamlessly throughout your day. Moreover, experts in the field of behavior modification state with certainty that a slip here and there is part of the behavior change process. This we do know, to establish and protect your healthy boundaries requires will power, assertiveness, high self-esteem and some good time management skills. Here is a closer look at each.

1. Will Power: There Is A Way!

Will power is the unique alchemy of motivation, inspiration and self-control. It is as much taking action toward a goal as it is inaction; preventing yourself from doing something you might later regret. Research on willpower and self-control underscores the importance of positive self-talk, also known as "positive affirmations." Common sense reminds us that negative self-talk (ego fear-based thinking) becomes self-defeating. It was will power that empowered civil rights activist Rosa Parks to take her seat on that bus in Alabama. It's also will power that enables you to go out and exercise or turn off the laptop or smart phone and spend some quality time with your family. It's important to remember that guilt only decreases will power. So, if you find that tomorrow your will power is weak, don't beat yourself up. Start where you are and progress from there. Exercise 2.4 *Damn, I'm Good!* outlines a strategy for using positive affirmations to strengthen your sense of will power. Good luck, you can do it!

2. Creative Assertiveness

In simple terms there are three types of behaviors; 1) Passive; being walked over (this promotes feelings of victimization, hence not recommended). 2) Aggressive; walking over people (also known as bullying and NOT recommended). 3) Assertive; holding your ground, diplomatically. When it comes to creating healthy boundaries, the clear choice is the assertive path. To be assertive means to be firm, but polite. It means communicating your boundaries, and not swaying to criticism when others (those who demonstrate passive or aggressive

> *Practice and more practice is the key until it becomes a routine woven seamlessly throughout your day.*

behaviors) mock you for holding your own ground. Being assertive means being empowered to say, "No" if saying "Yes" means violating a healthy boundary or promotes feelings of victimization. Learning to say no politely takes practice— sometimes lots of practice. Being successful with your healthy boundaries will take assertiveness. And there will be those people (like little children) who will test your boundaries, sometimes to no end. Be flexible, but hold strong.

3. Giving Self-Esteem A Boost!

Will power is important to maintaining healthy boundaries, but self-esteem is equally essential. In a stress-filled world overflowing with negativity, having a deflated sense of self-worth is all too common. Moreover, the advertising industry is great at making everyone feel insecure about their weight, hair, social status and other aspects too numerous to mention, yet equally bothersome. Self-esteem is more than just a sense of self-worth. Like will power, self-esteem is a unique alchemy of confidence, courage, humbleness and self-acceptance. Experts in the field of psychology have noted that five aspects of self-esteem are essential to promote a healthy life. They include: healthy role models, a sense of uniqueness, a sense of empowerment, a strong social support group and calculated risk-taking. While levels of self-esteem can fluctuate from day to day, there are some simple ways to boost your self-esteem. In doing so, you strengthen your center of gravity to withstand the prevailing winds of uncertainty, and become resilient should you slip and fall. Remember, there is a fine line between being perceived as confident and arrogant. Choose your behaviors wisely. Exercise 2.5, *Boosting Your Self-Esteem* invites you to explore the aspects of self-esteem in more detail, and steers you in the direction of a good boost!

4. Time Management

There is a funny proverb that states, "When all is said and done, there is a lot more said, than done." The fourth component of healthy boundaries involves making the time to practice your healthy boundaries. Many of our best intentions never see the light of day because we don't make the time to commit to a new schedule of healthy behaviors. As the expression goes, "To know and not to do, is not to know."

Today, we find ourselves living in a culture of distractions where making quality time to do things is greatly compromised. An abundance of choices and options is great, but it can also be overwhelming and quite distracting. And as great as all of our technology gadgets are, they can also become time robbers (e.g., searching Google for one thing can easily become an hour of web surfing). If you are like most people, most likely you are feeling some sense of time-crunch these days. The topic of time management is quite extensive, yet the basics are essential to acknowledge with regard to establishing healthy boundaries. If we don't make the time, our best intentions go to waste. To get a better sense if you are feeling the squeeze, consider completing the survey in Exercise 2.6, *Time Crunch Questionnaire* as an awareness

"when all is said and done, there is a lot more said, than done."

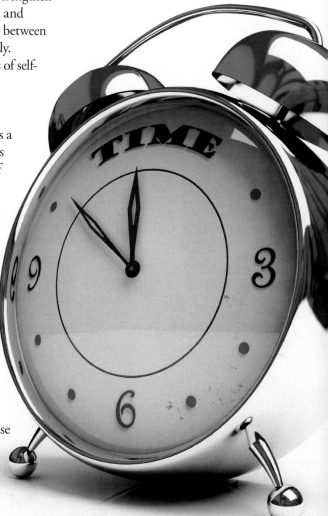

> "The road to the "Good Life" may have a few potholes and detours, but it also has some amazing vistas, rest stops and plenty of roadside attractions, all of which are worth experiencing."

tool to help calibrate your mind for new and improved healthy boundaries. In no uncertain terms, time management has become more than simply making a list of things to do. It now includes removing and deleting things that steal your precious time. Exercise 2.7, *Practicing The Art of Subtraction* invites you to examine the things in your life that may need to be edited out.

Without a doubt, healthy boundaries are essential for a healthy life; the good life. The following is a quote from a colleague who recently took some time to implement a few healthy boundaries in his life. In his words:

I was blessed with a pretty good life, but like most people I took it for granted. Some might say I lived on the edge. I lived by the expression, "If you are not living on the edge, you are taking up too much room." The only problem with living on the edge (as long as I did) is you can fall off, crash and ultimately hurt yourself, which I did. Some people call it rock bottom. I call it a face plant in reality. My world crumbled (over a period of several years, actually) and I could barely find the pieces to put myself back together. But I did. Slowly. One day at a time, one piece at a time. I have learned to become resilient. Today I eat less, exercise more and get a lot more sleep. I spend less time in virtual reality and more time in actual reality. I have a lot fewer friends, but better quality friends. I've learned that you can say "no" and people will still like you. I have also learned that it's true that everything works best in moderation. Life isn't a sprint. It's more like an ultra-marathon relay. It's essential to pace yourself. At 40 years old, I have learned to pace myself. In doing so, I have learned that I can enjoy life today with the promise that I will be around tomorrow. If I can learn this lesson, anyone can. My life isn't perfect, but whose is?! What I can say today is that my life is excellent, and you cannot ask for more than that.

The road to the "good life" may have a few potholes and detours, but it also has some amazing vistas, rest stops and plenty of roadside attractions, all of which are worth experiencing. The following exercises are intended to help you gain some awareness around some specific habits and behaviors that might need a little grooming. The following chapters explore the four basic components of wellness in more detail. Within each chapter you will find additional exercises, surveys, questionnaires and awareness tools that will help serve as a guide for healthy optimal living.

[EXERCISE 2.1]

Creating Healthy Boundaries

We are living in an age in which the average person has very poor boundaries in his or her life. Technology may be a factor, but it's not the only reason. People bring their work home while at the same time problems from home invade their professional lives. It seems that almost everyone has poor financial boundaries, with the average person carrying well over $5,000 annually in credit card debt. People think nothing of bringing their cell phones into restaurants and movie theaters, and what begins as just an hour in front of the television ends up being an entire evening. Poor personal boundaries result in feelings of being overwhelmed, annoyed and victimized—all of which contribute to a critical mass of stress.

Healthy boundaries require an insight about what's appropriate in each and every setting in which you find yourself. In essence, you need to discover what boundaries you need to create to maintain a sense of personal balance. Next, healthy boundaries require courage to assert your boundaries so that they are not violated. Finally, healthy boundaries require willpower and discipline so that you can establish better structure and stability in your life.

I. List four areas in your life that you feel have weak boundaries (or perhaps no boundaries). Examples might include finances, alcohol, technology, or television watching.

1. _____
   _____
2. _____
   _____
3. _____
   _____
4. _____
   _____

II. Now, list four healthy boundaries that you would like to create in your life to bring about a sense of balance. Then add a few words about what you can do to have these boundaries honored.

1. _____
   _____
2. _____
   _____
3. _____
   _____
4. _____
   _____

[EXERCISE 2.2]

Master Or Slave: The Internet Addiction Survey

A new social addiction has appeared on the scene, and it has ruined friendships, marriages, grade point averages and boardroom meetings. By some accounts, the Internet, Facebook updates, text messaging, emails, YouTube, Skype, Pinterest, video games, gambling, Instagram, Wikipedia, and online shopping have magnified the human need of acceptance; the need to feel needed. Eating is a basic human drive, but a food addiction is problematic. Like eating, access to the Internet as a public utility has become a part of everyday life, yet like a powerful black hole, one can become lost to the point of derailing one's life and those in one's immediate orbit including family, friends and co-workers. Are you a master or slave to the Internet? The following questionnaire may help you answer this question.

1 = Rarely/Never   2 = Occasionally   3 = Frequently   4 = Often   5 = Nearly Always

#		
1.	One of the first things I do each morning is go online to check text messages, emails, Facebook updates or other websites of interest.	
2.	Even though I might just check in briefly with social media sites, I end up online for a lot longer than I plan, sometimes for hours.	
3.	Although it might be considered illegal, I have been known to text while driving.	
4.	I check Facebook or Google Plus comments and emails several times an hour each day.	
5.	I become fidgety when I cannot pull out my smart phone or iPad and get online to check messages, text messages, or social media updates.	
6.	It's quite common for me to pull out my smart phone or tablet during a conversation with friends and check something online… then quickly check favorite social media sites.	
7.	I post updates on Facebook and then repeatedly check to see who "likes" and comments on what I post, as well as frequently comment on other postings.	
8.	I am easily distracted surfing the Internet, sometimes forgetting what I originally went online for.	
9.	I begin to feel agitated, perhaps even depressed when I don't have access to my smart phone (e.g., dead battery, dead zone, etc.) for long periods of time.	
10.	In the course of a typical day, I end up spending more time online than real-time contact with friends, family and peers.	
11.	I tend to get aggravated when I get interrupted while online.	
12.	Online activities have a priority over work and many home responsibilities.	
13.	Life without social networking, texting and web-surfing would be extremely boring, even unhappy for me.	
14.	I quickly check email, Facebook or other social networking sites before meetings, appointments, etc.	
15.	I have a hard time turning my cell phone/smart phone off.	
16.	Friends and family comment about my online use.	
17.	I become defensive when people comment on my use of the Internet.	
18.	My sleep time has decreased since smart phones, tablets etc. have come into my life.	
19.	I watch TV, listen to the radio or do other things while online.	
20.	The last thing I do before I go to sleep is check text messages and social media site updates.	

TOTAL SCORE ❯

Key: Score your answers by adding the points for each question for a grand total. The higher your score, the greater your level of addiction and the issues and concerns associated with Internet use or what is now commonly called, screen addictions.

Please use the following scale to help measure your score.

SCORE

10-39 points = Indicates normal online use. Keep in mind that normal is not always healthy.

40-69 points = Indicates that your Internet activity leans in the direction of Internet addiction and healthy boundaries with Internet use are a good idea.

70-100 points = Indicates that the amount of time you spend online is associated with addictive behaviors and thought should be given to changing this behavior with the creation and practice of strong healthy boundaries.

[EXERCISE 2.3]

Cheese With Your Whine? A Healthy Catharsis

First and foremost remember this: It is OK to whine… just not all the time! As the saying goes, "You can visit Pity City, you just can't live there." But boy do people try! Simply stated, whining is cathartic; it's a healthy emotional release. But just like you wouldn't sit on the toilet all day (that's another kind of release) neither should you whine all day, every day. This exercise invites you to put a healthy boundary on whining. Keeping in mind the premise of balance, the first half of this exercise invites you to whine, followed by the second part that invites you to empower yourself with a different (positive) perspective. Some people may call this the Pollyanna—rose-colored glasses view, but in truth, it offers perspective to what can become a myopic view of your life. As the expression goes, "Every situation has a good side and a bad side. Each moment you decide."

PART 1: Write down a problem, concern, issue or dilemma that you are facing; feel free to complain. Explain how this makes you feel. Then explain your expectation of how things should be or how you wish they were.

_____

_____

_____

_____

_____

_____

_____

_____

PART 2: There is always a positive side to a bad situation. Always! It's time to put on some rose-colored glasses and take a different perspective. Using the same issue or problem you used in Part I, take a moment to write down something positive about this bad experience, even if it's that you have learned never to do it again.

_____

_____

_____

_____

_____

_____

_____

_____

[EXERCISE 2.4]

Damn, I'm Good! Positive Affirmation Statements

Positive affirmation statements are thoughts or expressions that you can repeat to yourself to boost your self-esteem. These words of inspiration highlight the positive aspects of your personality traits and characteristics that enhance and nurture your self-esteem. They are expressions that build your confidence, provide inspiration, lift the human spirit to rise above mediocrity, and help you function at your highest human potential. Olympic swimming champion Michael Phelps uses positive affirmation statements to will his cache of gold medals. Mountain climber Joe Simpson credited the use of positive affirmations with saving his life from a near lethal accident. Nelson Mandela's affirmation statement became the famous poem Invictus.

It is easy to give yourself negative feedback about almost anything. We each have a critic (the ego) who metaphorically sits on our shoulder and whispers negative thoughts in our ear. The media does this too, striking at our insecurities through subliminal and overt advertising with over 1,500 messages a day. In addition, we often interpret feedback to be negative from family, friends and other people who pass in and out of our lives. But worst of all, perhaps as a learned behavior, we continually feed ourselves negative thoughts which continually deflate (and sabotage) our self-esteem.

Although there are no specific rules, there are some guidelines that can make your positive affirmations work best for you:

Your Affirmation Statement(s):

_____

_____

_____

_____

_____

_____

_____

_____

_____

_____

_____

Finally, you can always do what my friend Zach does. He simply says, "Healthy boundaries" when he wants to pull the reins in… good advice!

[EXERCISE 2.5]

Giving Your Self-Esteem A Healthy Boost

Self-esteem is thought to be comprised of five components: Uniqueness, Role Models, Empowerment, Connectedness, and Calculated Risk-Taking. With this in mind, let's take a look at your level of self-esteem with respect to these five areas. Try to answer the following questions as best as you can.

I. Uniqueness: **List five characteristics or personal attributes that make you feel special and unique (e. g., sense of humor, being a good cook, a passion for travel):**

1. _____
2. _____
3. _____
4. _____
5. _____

II. Empowerment: **List five areas or aspects of your life in which you feel you are empowered:**

1. _____
2. _____
3. _____
4. _____
5. _____

III. Mentors & Role Models: **Name five people (heroes, mentors, or role models) who have one or more characteristics that you admire and wish to emulate or enhance as a part of your own personality. Please describe the person and what trait or traits they possess.**

1. _____
2. _____
3. _____
4. _____
5. _____

IV. Connectedness: Friends and family are now thought to be crucial to one's health status. To have a sense of belonging is very important in one's life. Who (or what) gives you a sense of belonging? Please describe each in a sentence.

1. _____
2. _____
3. _____
4. _____
5. _____

V. Calculated Risk-Taking: List five good risks that you have taken in the past year that you feel have augmented your sense of self-worth and courage.

1. _____
2. _____
3. _____
4. _____
5. _____

[EXERCISE 2.6]

The Time-Crunch Questionnaire

Please answer the following questions as you are (not how you would like to be) regarding your time management skills. Add up the numbers you circled and check the questionnaire key to determine your level of time management skills.

		1 = Rarely	**2 = Sometimes**	**3 = Often**			
1.	I tend to procrastinate with projects and responsibilities				1	2	3
2.	My bedtime varies upon the workload I have each day				1	2	3
3.	I am the kind of person who leaves things until the last minute				1	2	3
4.	I forget to make or refer to "to do" lists to keep me organized				1	2	3
5.	I spend more than two hours watching television each night				1	2	3
6.	I tend to have multiple projects going on at the same time				1	2	3
7.	I tend to put work ahead of family and friends				1	2	3
8.	My life seems to be full of endless interruptions and distractions				1	2	3
9.	I tend to spend a lot of time on the phone talking to friends				1	2	3
10.	Multi-tasking is my middle name. I am a great multi-tasker				1	2	3
11.	My biggest problem with time management is prioritization				1	2	3
12.	I am a perfectionist when it comes to getting things done				1	2	3
13.	I never seem to have enough time for my personal life				1	2	3
14.	I tend to set unrealistic goals to accomplish tasks				1	2	3
15.	I reward myself *before* getting things done on time				1	2	3
16.	I just never have enough hours in the day to get things done				1	2	3
17.	I can spend untold hours distracted while surfing the Internet				1	2	3
18.	I tend to not trust others to get things done when I can do it better myself				1	2	3
19.	If I am completely honest, I tend to be a workaholic				1	2	3
20.	I have been known to skip meals in order to complete projects				1	2	3
21.	I will clean my room, garage, or kitchen before I really get to work on projects				1	2	3
22.	I will often help friends with their work before doing my own				1	2	3
23.	I tend to spend time on less important, but more satisfying things at the cost of being efficient				1	2	3
24.	I end up wasting a lot of time with technology and gadgets				1	2	3
25.	I often find it hard to get motivated to get things done				1	2	3

SCORES ❯

TOTAL SCORE ❯

SCORE

75-51 points = Poor time management skills (time to re-evaluate your life skills)
50-26 points = Fair time management skills (time to pull in the reins a bit)
0-25 points = Excellent time management skills (keep doing what you are doing!)

[EXERCISE 2.7]

Practicing The Art Of Subtraction

Does your life feel cluttered with too much stuff? Is your garage and basement filled with stuff that you haven't used or seen in years? Are there people in your life who are so emotionally needy that when you see them, you want to run and hide? Are there things in your life that at first seemed to simplify things and now they seem to be complicating things? If so, you might want to consider engaging in the Art of Subtraction (also known as editing your life). Please read through these items and answer the questions to help identify where you need to pull the reins in so that you don't feel victimized by your own behaviors.

I. Clutter: **Walk through your house or apartment and make a list of five things that fall in the category of personal clutter (this can include equipment, clothes, books, or anything lying on the floor). Once you have made this list, collect the things and consider giving them away to the Goodwill or some other charitable organization.**

1. _____
2. _____
3. _____
4. _____
5. _____

II. People: **Are there people in your life who take up time rather than contribute to your quality of life? Take inventory if you have any "friends" who seem to be a drain on your emotional energy. The next question to ask yourself is: Do you drain other people's energy? Do you give as well as take in your relationships and friendships?**

1. _____
2. _____
3. _____
4. _____
5. _____

III. Simplicity vs. Complexity: **We tend to bring things into our lives out of both interest and fear. What things are in your life right now that may have begun out of interest, but now you are ready to let go of? Another way to phrase this question is to ask yourself: What things in your life tend to add complexity rather than simplicity? Once you have identified three things, begin to ask yourself what you can do to subtract these things to bring your life back into balance.**

1. _____
2. _____
3. _____
4. _____
5. _____

[CHAPTER 3]

Physical Well-Being

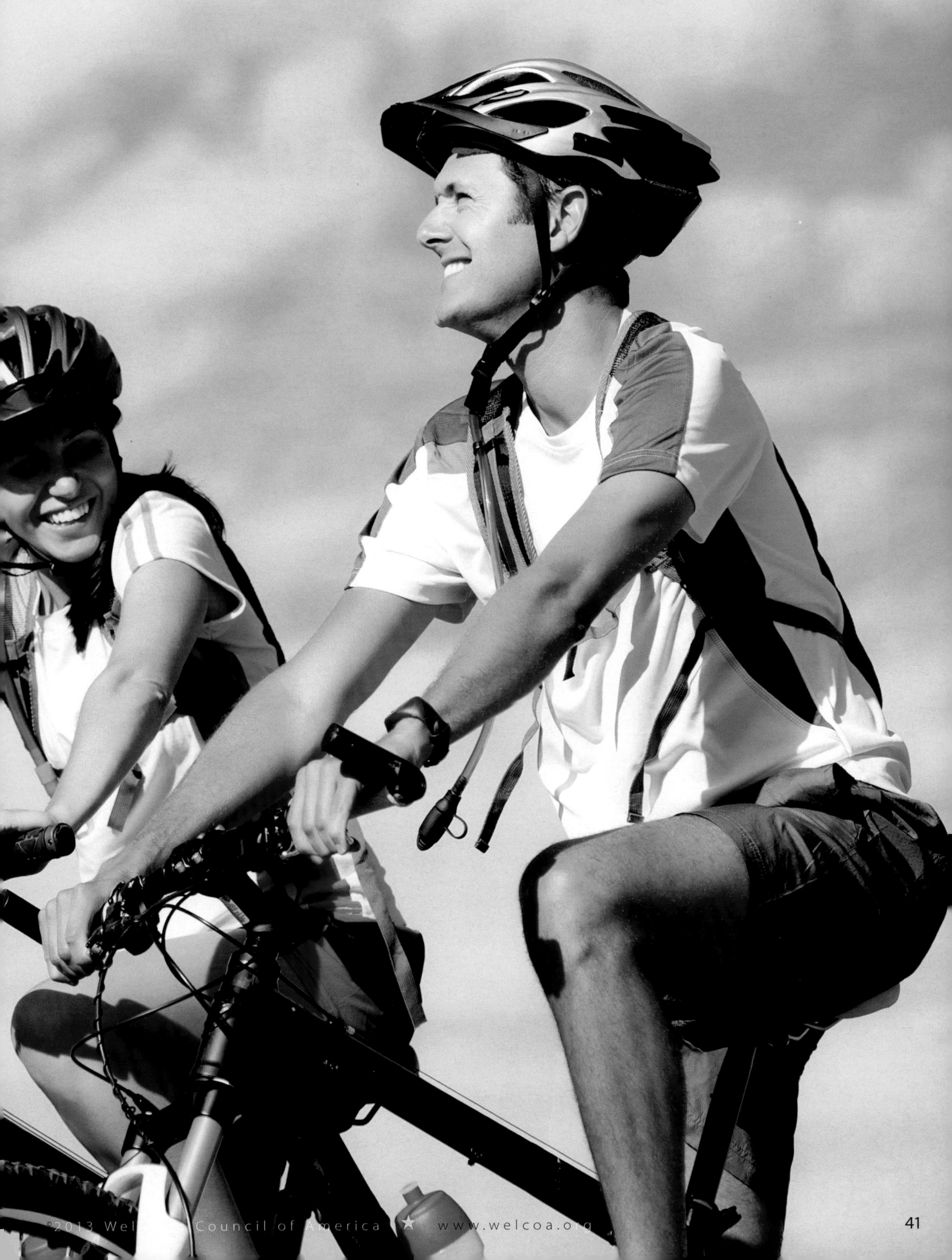

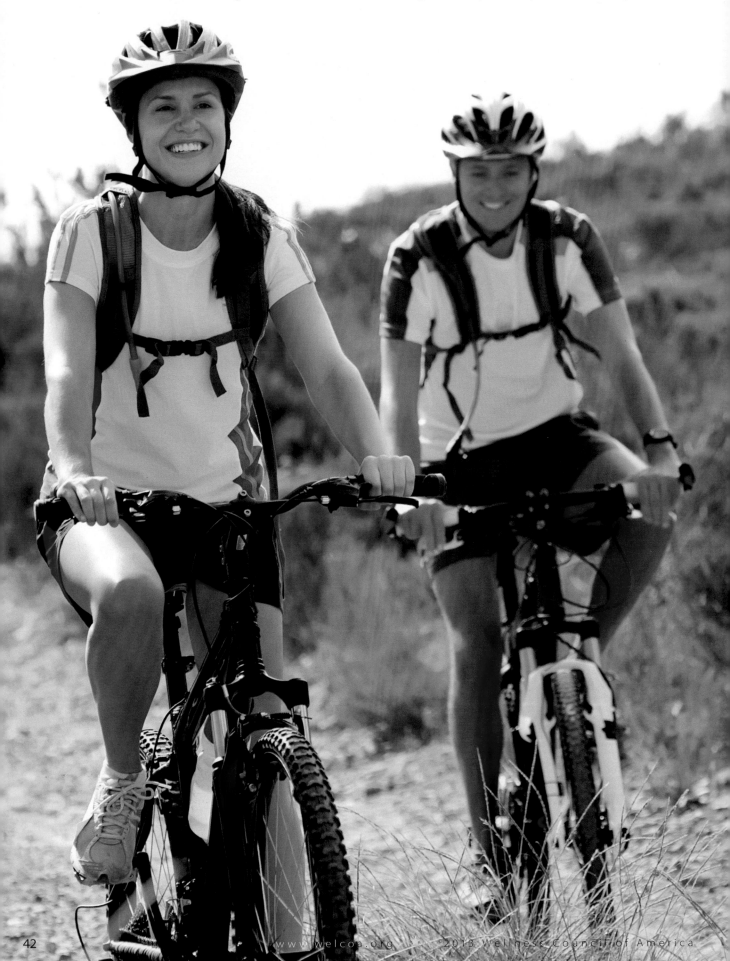

[CHAPTER 3]

Physical Well-Being

O f the four primary components of wellness, physical well-being has held the limelight for centuries. The reason is obvious. It's the easiest to measure; height, weight, resting heart rate and blood pressure, HDL and LDL serum levels, even bone density, to name a few. For this reason, over the years most wellness programs have placed the greatest emphasis on this specific wellness component. When corporate wellness programs first began in the 1970s, the biggest health issue at that time was coronary heart disease. As a result, the emphasis of wellness programming was placed on improving the cardiovascular system to prevent heart attacks and strokes. Back then most wellness programs were primarily fitness classes involving aerobic training with jogging and walking programs. Today, cardiovascular disease shares the health headlines with several other chronic diseases including cancer, diabetes, obesity and a score of autoimmune diseases (e.g., lupus, rheumatoid arthritis, fibromyalgia, Crohn's disease, multiple sclerosis, etc.)

Indeed, cardiovascular fitness is important, but your body has seven other essential physiological systems (i.e., musculoskeletal, nervous, respiratory, digestive, reproductive, endocrine and immune/lymphatic system) that also need attention. Together these physiological systems act as an alliance for optimal health and well-being. So connected are these systems that when one is compromised, all the rest will suffer. As mentioned in the first chapter,

> "Together these physiological systems act as an alliance for optimal health and well-being."

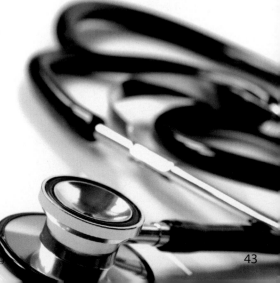

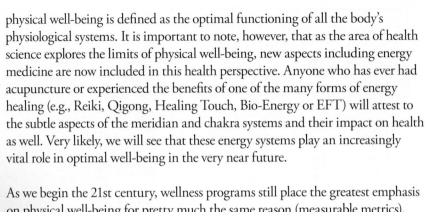

physical well-being is defined as the optimal functioning of all the body's physiological systems. It is important to note, however, that as the area of health science explores the limits of physical well-being, new aspects including energy medicine are now included in this health perspective. Anyone who has ever had acupuncture or experienced the benefits of one of the many forms of energy healing (e.g., Reiki, Qigong, Healing Touch, Bio-Energy or EFT) will attest to the subtle aspects of the meridian and chakra systems and their impact on health as well. Very likely, we will see that these energy systems play an increasingly vital role in optimal well-being in the very near future.

As we begin the 21st century, wellness programs still place the greatest emphasis on physical well-being for pretty much the same reason (measurable metrics). However, depending on the wellness program and staff of experts, attention is also placed on the musculoskeletal system, digestive system (nutrition) and sometimes the immune system depending on the quality of stress management offerings. For example, classes in Hatha Yoga, Tai Chi, healthy back and mindfulness meditation continue to round out the wellness offerings to promote physical well-being. And as noted in Chapter One, attention to physical well-being impacts one's mental, emotional and spiritual well-being as well.

Take Good Care Of Your Body

Renowned inventor and philosopher, Buckminster Fuller, once said that the human body is our one and only space suit in which to inhabit planet earth. It comes with its own set of oxygen tanks (lungs), metabolic waste removal system (GI tract), a sensory detector system to enjoy all the pleasures for planetary exploration and an immune defense system to ensure the health of the space suit in the occasional harsh global environments. The human body is quite remarkable; however, caution is noted to pay as much attention to the internal structure as well as the outward appearance. Additionally, this specially designed space suit is also equipped with a unique program for self-healing. Factors associated with this self-healing process include the basic common health behaviors associated with longevity: regular physical exercise, proper nutrition, adequate sleep, the avoidance of cigarettes and drugs (and other toxic chemicals) and a supportive community of friends and family. This chapter explores these aspects of self-healing, more commonly known as healthy lifestyle habits for physical well-being.

Your Remarkable Body!

How well do your know your body? Sure, you might know the values of your height, weight, resting blood pressure and heart rate, as well as your serum cholesterol levels. You might even know your values for bone density. But did you know that your body makes new blood cells every 28 days? The cells of your skin are replaced every 30 days. Estimates suggest that new cells are constantly being created in various parts of our bodies over specific periods so that every seven years we have a completely new body. People who quit smoking will see their lungs return to "normal" within 14 years, and many people have donated part of their liver to family members knowing that their own liver will regenerate itself in less than six months' time. Your body is simply amazing! And although your body is not a machine, this metaphor comes in handy with regard to regular maintenance. All things being equal, the human body strives for a healthy state, despite poor exercise, sleep and eating habits. All attempts to strive for a healthy state becomes at odds with the aging process, making good exercise, sleep and eating habits all the more important after age 30. How is your picture of health? Exercise 3.1 offers you a quick look by taking an inventory of your health status.

Good physical well-being habits are common sense, but in this day of rapid change, techno-stress and increasing responsibilities, common sense is not too common. Here is a quick review to help you recalibrate your habits for physical well-being.

Healthy Habits For Exercise And Physical Activity

If you take a look at the news today, it's hard not to notice our love affair with youth and beauty: Botox injections, liposuction, facelifts, tummy tucks and implants to name a few. Everyone is looking for a quick trip to the fountain of youth, yet there are no quick fixes or magic bullets for optimal health. Wait. There is one, kind of. It's called physical exercise. If you take the time to review the data on the beneficial effects of physical exercise, it reads like a how-to manual for drinking from the *Fountain of Youth*. Yet, rather than an immediate fix, the research is quite clear: The benefits of regular physical exercise take about six to eight weeks to appear, yet the investment in your health will be invaluable. There is no doubt that exercise dramatically slows the aging process. Moreover, it adds tremendous quality to your life. Here is a short list of these benefits:

> Decreased resting heart rate (improved heart function)
> Decreased resting blood pressure (improved heart function)
> Decreased body fat (improved figure)
> Increased bone density (stronger bones and joints)
> Decreased serum lipid levels (LDLs)
> Increased quality of sleep
> Increased immune system function

> Everyone is looking for a quick trip to the fountain of youth, yet there are no quick fixes or magic bullets for optimal health.

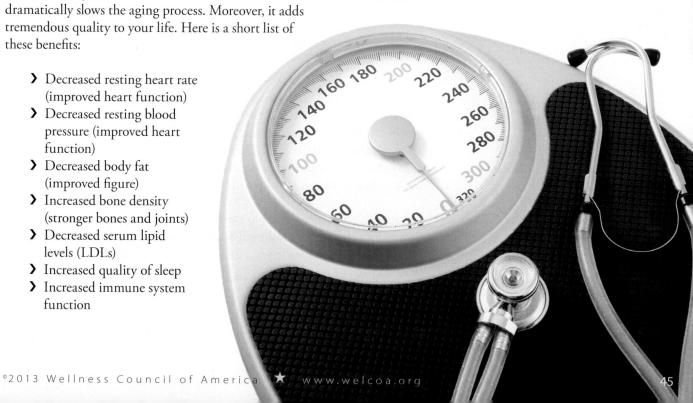

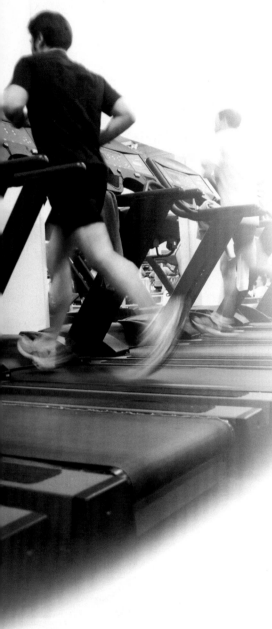

Stress And Disease: Fight Or Flight With A Bite

The human body may crave rest and relaxation, but truth be told, it also craves excitement; physical stimulation in the form of physical activity and exercise. The human body was created for motion, and for the most part, in our early years we do it quite well. As we get older, however, we find a million and one reasons not to exercise. The end result is a great physiological imbalance that often sets the stage for disease and illness. Engaging in a regular fitness program (even if it's just walking a few miles a day at sunset) is essential to achieving and maintaining the good life. A simple exercise program brings the body back into balance—back into homeostasis.

Research in the field of psychoneuroimmunology (PNI, or more commonly known as mind-body studies) reveals that the association between stress and disease is colossal, everything from the common cold to cancer to herpes to hemorrhoids. Exercise 3.2 invites you to do a quick check on your health through the lens of stress and disease. Stress may begin in the mind (as a perceived threat, coupled with an emotion of anger or fear) but thoughts and emotions quickly become neurotransmitter activity in the brain, which then cascades down through the hormonal system to sound the "fight or flight" response. When stress is left unresolved, the body becomes the battlefield for the war games of the mind. Exercise may be considered a stress to the body, but the good news is that it restores the body back to homeostasis through the parasympathetic rebound effect.

Components Of Fitness

Cardiovascular fitness is but one of several fitness components. Others include muscular strength (lifting a heavy object, like a suitcase), muscular endurance (carrying a heavy object like groceries a few blocks home), flexibility, agility and balance. Remember that a well-designed fitness program tries to include as many of these components as possible. Research also reveals that for the best results one must follow some simple yet specific guidelines called the All or None Principle of Exercise.

The All Or None Principle Of Exercise

The All or None exercise protocol for fitness is so well known today you can find it outlined on the back of cereal boxes. It can even be found woven into humorous birthday cards and late night television comedy routines. This protocol, also called the FITT Principle, means that all aspects must be fully engaged or none of the physiological benefits will appear. As the saying goes, use it or lose it. Let's review these dynamics once more:

Frequency: Frequency refers to the number of times per week you exercise. The magic number is a minimum of three times. You can exercise more often, but if you exercise fewer than three times per week, these beneficial changes become elusive.

> The human body was created for motion, and for the most part, in our early years we do it quite well.

Intensity: The activity must challenge the physiological system that is being worked (e.g., cardiovascular system, musculoskeletal system, etc.). Intensity is often measured in terms of one's target heart rate (75 percent of one's maximal heart rate) for cardiovascular endurance or pounds, reps and sets for weight lifting for muscular strength or muscular endurance.

Time (Duration): Exercise studies show that the minimum amount of time to work out is 20 minutes per session at the intensity that challenges the desired physiological system. When you add a proper warm–up and cool-down period (five minutes each) the minimum duration period equals about 30 minutes. You can exercise more, but again, less than 20 minutes won't help you attain the desired results. The anatomy of a workout includes a proper warm-up to allow for a proper redistribution of blood flow (from your body's core to the working muscles of the extremities).

Type Of Exercise: There are countless types of exercise and each specifically addresses one or more of the components of fitness. Walking, jogging and swimming are great for cardiovascular fitness. Weight training is ideal to improve levels of muscular strength and endurance. Yoga is considered wonderful to improve one's flexibility. The type of exercise you select should match your fitness goals to elicit the best response.

Energy Balance: Given the obesity epidemic in our culture, it would be a gross oversight to talk about physical fitness without addressing the importance of energy expenditure: calories. The topic of calories (and calorie counting) comes and goes in popularity, but the ageless wisdom is important to remember. Basal Metabolic Rate (BMR) is a term used to describe the number of calories (energy) your body burns in a 24-hour period with little or no activity. The amount is roughly 2,000 calories. Exercise each day may add another 300 to 400 calories, depending on the type and how long you exercise. If the foods we eat per day contain more calories than we burn, then weight gain is certain to happen. Conversely, if we consume less calories than we burn, then weight loss will occur. It's this simple! What people often forget is that BMR tends to decrease with age, yet eating habits tend to remain the same (hence one more reason for weight gain). There are many aspects to the obesity issue which are far too complicated to include in this workbook, but suffice it to say that energy balance is an important aspect to consider in regard to physical well-being.

Creating an exercise routine isn't hard. You can start with a simple waking routine. Because many people insist they just don't have time to exercise, the default exercise plan is this: Just get outside and move. Exercise 3.3 will help you get started. As always, check with your physician for any precautions and recommendations. Wellness coaches and personal fitness trainers can be of assistance too. When all is said and done, never underestimate the power of a good walking program.

> The type of exercise you select should match your fitness goals to elicit the best response.

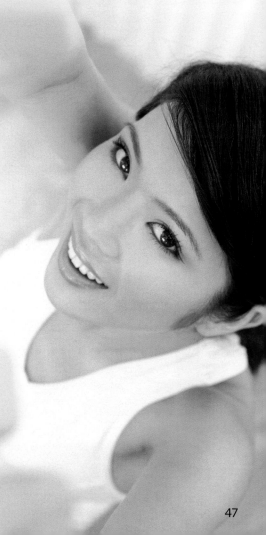

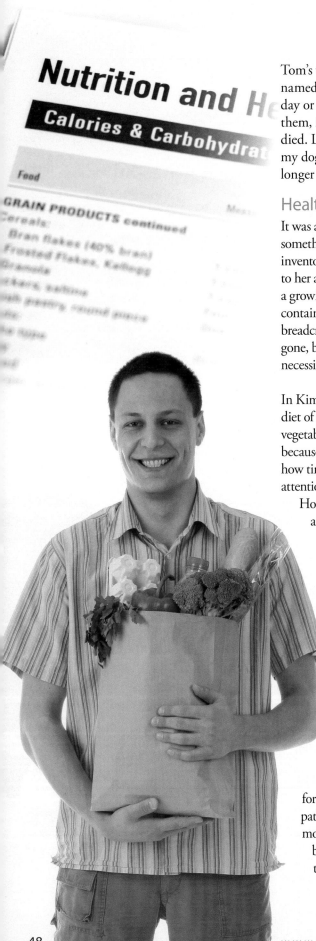

Tom's walking program started in earnest when he adopted a Siberian husky named Nome. "There is an expression I've heard with huskies: Walk each day or hell to pay. These dogs like to be exercised and it's not only good for them, it gets me out too. I bought this dog for companionship after my wife died. Little did I know just how healthy it would make me. Since walking my dog twice a day for the past six months, I have lost 10 pounds and no longer need my blood pressure medicine," Tom explained. "That's wellness!"

Healthy Habits For Good Nutrition

It was a large rash on Kim's hands and chest that first got her attention that something was wrong. After several visits to specialists and an exhaustive health inventory of several weeks leading up to the rash appearance, it was brought to her attention that perhaps she had a gluten intolerance. Kim is among a growing group of Americans with food allergies, specifically to all foods containing wheat, from the obvious (pasta) to the subtle (meatballs that contain breadcrumbs). Having removed all wheat products from her diet, the rash is now gone, but as Kim said, "It could come back at any time." For this reason, out of necessity, she has become quite vigilant about her eating habits.

In Kim's grandmother's day the basics of nutrition were simple: eat a balanced diet of carbohydrates, fats and proteins. Be sure to eat a variety of fruits and vegetables and drink plenty of water. Decades ago no one needed food labels because most foods came straight from the farm to the dinner plate. Boy, how times have changed in just a few generations. Today, people put as much attention to what is *not* in food as they do about what is in the food they eat. Hormones, antibiotics, pesticides, herbicides, and petrochemical fertilizers and genetically modified organisms are considered taboo. Terms like "organic," "free range," and "gluten-free" are now household words. In addition to all the anxiety about toxic food additives and preservatives is the concern about increased fat, sugar, salt and caffeine in our foods and the proliferation of fast foods, processed foods, junk foods and comfort foods (all of which are known as empty calories) in the standard American diet.

Suggestions For Healthy Eating

The first rule of good nutritional habits is not to feel guilty about what you typically eat or drink. Guilt is a poor motivator for changing behaviors, and in fact tends to backfire. So don't feel guilty about previous habits. Instead, become empowered to make a few simple changes to your diet that enhance the integrity of your immune system. Rather than create a guilt-ridden list of do's and don'ts for weight management, I would like to share some suggestions for maintaining the integrity of your immune system that contribute to your path to the good life. There is an old proverb from Hippocrates, the father of modern medicine, that states, "Let food be your medicine and let medicine be your food." Unfortunately today, rather than eating food as medicine, the vast majority of people eat food as poison (petrochemical fertilizers, antibiotics, hormones, etc.). Like toxins dumped into a river, the human body can only take so much before signs of disease and illness manifest. The following is a list of suggestions to tip the scale back to balance and promote a sense of optimal health and well-being.

1. Consume a good supply of antioxidants (beta carotene, vitamins C, E and selenium). These fight the damage of free radicals (oxygen molecules) which destroy cell membranes, DNA, RNA and mitochondria. Anti-oxidants can be found in fresh fruits and veggies.

2. Consume a good supply of fiber (30-40 grams/day with organic fruits and vegetables). Fiber helps clean the colon of toxic materials that might otherwise be absorbed into the bloodstream (colon cancer is the second leading cause of cancer in both men and women).

3. Drink plenty of fresh clean (filtered) water (a good goal is nearly clear urine). Water not only keeps you hydrated, but it also helps flush toxins out of your system.

4. Eat organic foods whenever possible. Organic foods are foods grown in soil clean of herbicides, pesticides, fungicides and petrochemical fertilizers which are now known to act as endocrine-mimickers, causing an imbalance with the regulation of hormones.

5. Consume foods in the rainbow diet (red, orange, yellow, green, blue and purple). This translates to: Eat a variety of fresh fruits and vegetables. Bioflavonoids, the substances responsible for food colors in fruits and veggies, are now known to help prevent cancer. Exercise 3.5 offers a quick look at the colors of foods and provides a ready-made list for the next time you are at the grocery store.

6. Consume a good supply and balance of Omega 3's (cold water fish and flax seed oil) and Omega 6s (vegetable oils). The body cannot produce some oils; hence it needs these from outside sources for everything from myelin sheaths around nerve cells to the formation of cell membranes to the creation of many hormones.

7. Watch and reduce your sugar intake. Sugar is now known to decrease the count of white blood cells in your body, making you more vulnerable to colds, flus and possibly cancer. It's always a good idea to reduce refined sugar in one's diet and high fructose corn syrup in one's diet.

Let food be your medicine and let medicine be your food.

> *If there is one rule to remember while eating it might be this: Eat one meal a day for your immune system.*

8. Decrease your intake of saturated fats (meat and dairy products). In the digestion process, fats have to first travel via the lymphatic system before they arrive in the liver. A diet high in fats taxes the immune system of which the lymphatic system is a big part.

9. Decrease/avoid trans-fatty acids (partially-hydrogenated oils). Trans-fats act like free radicals destroying the integrity of the cell membrane, RNA, DNA and cell mitochondria. Not only does this speed up the aging process, some experts suggest that trans-fats are associated with the pathology of coronary heart disease and possibly cancer.

10. Prepare food in the best way possible. Many important nutrients are destroyed in the process of cooking, often leaving meals with a deficient supply of vitamins and minerals. Fresh veggies are best prepared steamed (when soaked in water, the nutrients are leached out and then thrown down the drain). Experts also suggest that you avoid microwave ovens, as intense heat can also destroy nutrients.

Eating habits can also be greatly influenced by one's stress levels. When people are stressed they tend to be short on time to prepare foods, hence resort to foods that are easily accessible, such as fast foods and comfort foods. Not only are these foods loaded with sugar, salt and fats (which is why they taste so good), they are void of any vitamins and minerals needed for the healthy maintenance of your body. Exercise 3.4 is a survey that invites you to examine your eating habits and see if they might be influenced by your levels of stress. If there is one rule to remember with eating it might be this: Eat one meal a day for your immune system.

Healthy Habits for a Good Night's Sleep

According to a recent survey by the National Sleep Foundation, over 60 percent of Americans suffer from poor sleep quality resulting in everything from falling asleep on the job and absenteeism to marital problems and car accidents. A quick check of the nation's pulse reveals that insomnia, in all its many forms (transient, intermittent or chronic), has become one more in a growing list of national health epidemics. This health issue is evidenced with the proliferation of pharmaceutical ads promising the cure to the newest syndrome of the high tech age. Perhaps most troublesome is the dramatic incidence of insomnia reported in middle school and high school students whose brains are still developing. For adults and children alike, a succession of restless nights becomes a battle of thought processes between the conscious mind's inability to turn off and the unconscious mind's inability to communicate through dreams. The end result is that both sides claim casualties and neither side is victorious.

Insomnia is best defined as poor quality sleep, abnormal wakefulness, or the inability to sleep. Perhaps not surprisingly,

90 percent of those questioned in various surveys admit to emotional stress being the cause of their poor sleeping habits. Not only can stress (mental, emotional, physical or spiritual) affect quality and quantity of sleep, but the rebound effect of poor sleep can, in turn, affect one's stress levels making one become more irritable, apathetic, cynical, or anxious during normal waking hours. Left unresolved, the link between stress and insomnia can become a vicious unbroken cycle. While many people seek medical help and are often given a prescription for a quick fix, due to numerous side effects, drugs should be considered as a last resort (medications address symptoms, not causes). Conversely, many (if not all) techniques for stress management, including cardiovascular exercise, meditation, muscle massage, diaphragmatic breathing, Tai Chi and Hatha yoga have proven to be effective in promoting a good night's sleep by promoting mind-body-spirit homeostasis.

Sleep researchers have been studying various aspects of sleep in earnest for over half a century. Despite their best efforts they still come up empty handed when asked to fully explain the importance of sleep. Surely the body's physiology needs to restore itself, yet it appears that the mind needs time off even more so. Various studies reveal that people who are purposely deprived of this essential human drive show signs of psychosis—all of which reverses itself when full sleep patterns are restored. Some of the best research about sleep comes to us from the world of extreme sports where bicyclists who race across America (RAAM) have determined the minimal amount of sleep needed for peak performance is one complete REM (rapid eye movement) cycle, the last phase in an undisturbed two-hour segment where the mind moves from alpha waves to theta waves (in which REM is observed). While these extreme athletes have learned to lock in on this magic period, the coveted REM cycle seems ever elusive to millions of restless Americans tossing and turning all night. Dreams, which are known to occur mostly during REM cycles, also appear to be an essential factor for mental equilibrium during the waking hours of a busy day—even if you don't remember them.

Before the advent of electricity (and utility bills), it was believed that the average person slept a solid 10 hours each night. Sleep experts suggest that eight hours is the golden standard, yet they often confide that some people can excel on six hours while others would do best with the "pre-Edison" 10-hour quota. It appears that the real key to a good night's sleep is to get at least one (hopefully several) full cycles of REM/theta wave activity.

The Essence Of Good Sleep Hygiene

Sarah doesn't sleep well at night, and she hasn't for years. Over a cup of coffee and a few doughnuts she confides that it takes hours for her to fall asleep only to wake up several times in the course of the night, staring at the alarm clock wishing it was morning. Sarah is not alone in her quest for a good night's sleep

> *Left unresolved, the link between stress and insomnia can become a vicious unbroken cycle.*

> *America's addiction to coffee is as much a symptom as a possible cause of the problem.*

or better physical health. She has joined the ranks of millions of restless Americans who claim a similar disturbance in what should be a most pleasurable experience; one that we spend one-third of our lives engaged in. The rebound effect of poor quality sleep reveals itself in the normal waking hours through poor work productivity, irritability, anxiety, poor communication skills and several behaviors that are less than becoming to one's authentic self. America's addiction to coffee is as much a symptom as a possible cause of the problem. Insomnia has now been linked to weight gain and a compromised immune system as well. "My life would be perfect if I could gain a few more hours of sleep a night and lose a few pounds," Sarah said. She is not alone in this sentiment.

Stress plays a big role in the quality of sleep (or lack thereof) but there are many other aspects that contribute to what sleep experts call "sleep hygiene" also known as the ambiance of your bedroom. For example, room temperature plays a big role in the quality of sleep. Body core temperature drops in the evening hours as the body prepares to shut down in sleep mode. A room with an elevated temperature doesn't allow one's body core temp to do its job (note: this may explain the relationship between menopausal hot flashes and poor sleep quality). Secondly, good sleep hygiene requires darkness. Night-lights, bright alarm clock lights, full moon radiance as well as outside streetlights are all registered by the pineal gland, even when your eyes are shut, and this will affect the production and secretion of melatonin. Noise will certainly affect the quality of one's sleep hygiene as well. Noises include everything from your partner's snoring or teeth grinding to a blaring television, as well as pets self-grooming on the bed or street noise. Any of these disturbances that impede quality sleep is called "sleep stealers." Current research suggests that the number one sleep stealer is the television set in the bedroom. All aspects of good sleep hygiene require the recognition and enforcement of healthy boundaries. The following are some time-honored suggestions that when combined provide the ideal conditions for a good night's sleep.

Tips For Good Sleep Hygiene

1. Keep a regular sleep cycle. Make a habit of going to bed at the same time every night (within 15 minutes) and waking up at about the same time each morning (even weekends). You might also consider honoring your circadian rhythms by eating your dinner at approximately the same time each night. Many sleep experts note that one should not eat a big meal before falling asleep as this will interfere with one's sleep cycles (REM).

2. Create an ideal sleep ambience! Create a sleep friendly environment where bright lights, noise and all other sensory distractions are minimized, if not completely eliminated. Additionally, invest in a good bed and bedding. For a place in which people spend one-third of their lives, consider the best options to promote quality sleep. Remember, there is a good reason why the exclusive hotels around the world furnish their first class beds with Italian or Egyptian cotton sheets, down pillows and comforters. Start with a good mattress, but don't end there. Continue with a superior mattress pad, the highest quality sheets (higher thread counts equal a softness that lulls you into la-la land), and goose down pillows.

3. Eliminate TV before bed. Avoid watching television right before you go to bed. Instead, try reading to induce a sense of drowsiness. If your television is in your bedroom, move it out. If your children have a TV in their bedroom, do the same. If you cannot bear to remove your television, create healthy boundaries with your TV habits.

4. Stop using your cell phone after 6:00 p.m. One research study suggests that the microwaves radiating from cell phone use decreases the production of melatonin, the sleep hormone necessary for quality sleep. Moreover, extremely low frequency (ELF) vibrations are known to be a health hazard (just ask any policeman who uses a radar gun). It's best to curtail cell phone use hours before you plan to fall asleep. Once again, establish healthy boundaries with your cell phone.

5. Ensure that your bed is for sleeping only. In this 24/7 society, beds have become second home offices (e.g., balancing checkbooks, grading papers, reviewing taxes, etc.) Beds have also become recliners for watching TV and even a second dinner table. Good sleeping requires healthy boundaries. In this case, remove all non-sleep activities from your bedroom. Keep your bed as a vehicle for sleep (and sex) and leave it at that.

How good is your sleep hygiene? Exercise 3.6 offers a quick look at your current behaviors as an awareness tool for making a few changes to improve the quality of your sleep.

Circadian Rhythms And Physical Health

You may have heard the term "bio-rhythms", but the correct scientific term is called "circadian rhythms." From the Latin root "circa", which means about a day, the term circadian rhythms describes the various body rhythms in a 24-hour period. Simply stated, circadian rhythms are the body's internal clock. It is this clock that programs everything from the release of melatonin (the sleep hormone) in the evening to the regulation of the gastrointestinal tract. These rhythms are based on the earth's rotation and they have been ingrained in our DNA since the dawn of humanity. In today's world, they are every bit as important, yet often ignored, due to our love affair

> Make a habit of going to bed at the same time every night (within 15 minutes) and waking up at the same time each morning even weekends.

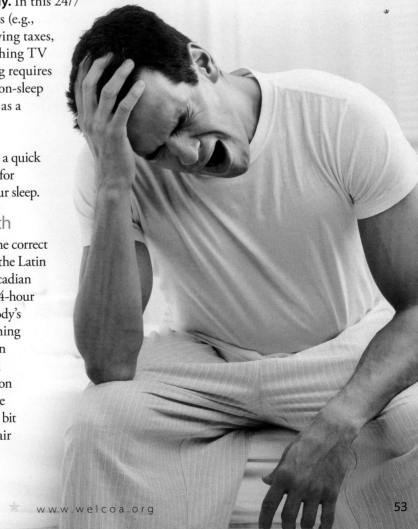

with technology (the use of artificial light, television, and an array of electrical devices such as smart phones and tablets are known to throw off these rhythms.) Research in the field of circadian rhythms suggests that our bodies do best when kept to a regular schedule with regard to sleep, meals and exercise. For example, eating breakfast, lunch and dinner at the same time each day, going to bed and waking up at the same time every day and exercising at approximately the same time every day. People who keep their body on a regular schedule and who are in tune with these rhythms tend to live longer, healthier lives.

Conversely, when we get off schedule, our body's physiology has a harder time adjusting to this form of stress. Over time, the end result is a greater propensity toward disease and illness as well as a more rapid aging process. Oncologists will tell you that cancer cells respond best to chemotherapy in the mid-morning hours as compared to early evening hours. Athletes will tell you that their best competitions are held at the same time as their practice workouts. The human body craves habitual routines. How are your daily routines? Exercise 3.7, *Circadian Rhythms* invites you to look at your life through the lens of a 24-hour clock and remind you of the importance of maintaining a well-tuned body clock.

Physical well-being is more than just eating broccoli and doing aerobics. It involves being mindful of all aspects of your physical health, from the vitality of your skin to the integrity of your immune system and everything in between. This chapter is but a brief introduction to the concepts of this wellness component. And as you will see each component is closely tied to the other three making for one dynamic health experience. And while it may be a bit overwhelming at times, the bottom line is to enjoy life to the fullest, in whatever capacity that may allow.

> "It involves being mindful of all aspects of your physical health, from the vitality of your skin to the integrity of your immune system and everything in between."

[EXERCISE 3.1]

Your Picture Of Health

We all have an idea of what ideal health is. Many of us take our health for granted until something goes wrong to remind us that the picture of health is compromised. Although health may seem to be objective, it will certainly vary from person to person over the aging process. The following questions are based on characteristics associated with longevity (none of which consider any genetic factors). Rather than answering the questions to see how long you may live, complete this inventory to determine your current picture of health.

	3 = Often	2 = Sometimes	1 = Rarely	0 = Never
1. With rare exception, I sleep on average 7 to 8 hours each night.	3	2	1	0
2. I tend to eat my meals at the same time each day.	3	2	1	0
3. I keep my bedtime consistent every night.	3	2	1	0
4. I do cardiovascular exercise at least three times per week.	3	2	1	0
5. My weight is considered ideal for my height.	3	2	1	0
6. Without exception, my alcohol consumption is in moderation.	3	2	1	0
7. I consider my nutritional habits to be exceptional.	3	2	1	0
8. My health status is considered excellent, with no pre-existing conditions.	3	2	1	0
9. I neither smoke, nor participate in the use of recreational drugs.	3	2	1	0
10. I have a solid group of friends with whom I socialize regularly.	3	2	1	0
SCORES ❯				

TOTAL SCORE ❯

SCORE

26-30 points = Excellent health habits   14-19 points = Questionable health habits

20-25 points = Moderate health habits   0-13 points = Poor health habits

[EXERCISE 3.2]

Physical Symptoms Questionnaire

Please look over this list of stress-related symptoms and circle how often they have occurred in the past week, how severe they seemed to you and how long they lasted. Then reflect on the past week's workload and see if you notice any connection.

		How Often? (number of days in the past week)								How Severe? (1 = mild, 5 = severe)					How Long? (1 = 1 hour, 5 = all day)				
1.	Tension headache	0	1	2	3	4	5	6	7	1	2	3	4	5	1	2	3	4	5
2.	Migraine headache	0	1	2	3	4	5	6	7	1	2	3	4	5	1	2	3	4	5
3.	Muscle tension (neck and/or shoulders)	0	1	2	3	4	5	6	7	1	2	3	4	5	1	2	3	4	5
4.	Muscle tension (lower back)	0	1	2	3	4	5	6	7	1	2	3	4	5	1	2	3	4	5
5.	Joint pain	0	1	2	3	4	5	6	7	1	2	3	4	5	1	2	3	4	5
6.	Cold	0	1	2	3	4	5	6	7	1	2	3	4	5	1	2	3	4	5
7.	Flu	0	1	2	3	4	5	6	7	1	2	3	4	5	1	2	3	4	5
8.	Stomachache	0	1	2	3	4	5	6	7	1	2	3	4	5	1	2	3	4	5
9.	Stomach/abdominal bloating/distention/gas	0	1	2	3	4	5	6	7	1	2	3	4	5	1	2	3	4	5
10.	Diarrhea	0	1	2	3	4	5	6	7	1	2	3	4	5	1	2	3	4	5
11.	Constipation	0	1	2	3	4	5	6	7	1	2	3	4	5	1	2	3	4	5
12.	Ulcer flare-up	0	1	2	3	4	5	6	7	1	2	3	4	5	1	2	3	4	5
13.	Asthma attack	0	1	2	3	4	5	6	7	1	2	3	4	5	1	2	3	4	5
14.	Allergies	0	1	2	3	4	5	6	7	1	2	3	4	5	1	2	3	4	5
15.	Canker/cold sores	0	1	2	3	4	5	6	7	1	2	3	4	5	1	2	3	4	5
16.	Dizzy spells	0	1	2	3	4	5	6	7	1	2	3	4	5	1	2	3	4	5
17.	Heart palpitations (racing heart)	0	1	2	3	4	5	6	7	1	2	3	4	5	1	2	3	4	5
18.	TMJ (temporormandibular joint)	0	1	2	3	4	5	6	7	1	2	3	4	5	1	2	3	4	5
19.	Insomnia	0	1	2	3	4	5	6	7	1	2	3	4	5	1	2	3	4	5
20.	Nightmares	0	1	2	3	4	5	6	7	1	2	3	4	5	1	2	3	4	5
21.	Fatigue	0	1	2	3	4	5	6	7	1	2	3	4	5	1	2	3	4	5
22.	Hemorrhoids	0	1	2	3	4	5	6	7	1	2	3	4	5	1	2	3	4	5
23.	Pimples/acne	0	1	2	3	4	5	6	7	1	2	3	4	5	1	2	3	4	5
24.	Cramps	0	1	2	3	4	5	6	7	1	2	3	4	5	1	2	3	4	5
25.	Frequent accidents	0	1	2	3	4	5	6	7	1	2	3	4	5	1	2	3	4	5
26.	Other (please specify) _____	0	1	2	3	4	5	6	7	1	2	3	4	5	1	2	3	4	5

TOTAL ❯ TOTAL ❯ TOTAL ❯

TOTAL SCORE ❯

SCORE

Look over the entire list. Do you observe any patterns or relationships between your stress levels and your physical health? A value over 30 points may indicate a stress-related health problem. If it seems that these symptoms are related to undue stress, they probably are. While medical treatment is advocated when necessary, the regular use of relaxation techniques may lessen the intensity, frequency and duration of these episodes.

[EXERCISE 3.3]

Creating An Exercise Program

To help you start (or maintain) your exercise routine, here are a few things to consider:

1. What is your favorite activity: _____

2. What time of day is best suited to spend 30 minutes for exercise: _____

3. Do you like to exercise alone or with a friend or two: _____

4. If you do like to exercise with friends, include their names here: _____

_____

5. What is your target heart rate? _____

   To determine your target heart rate follow this simple equation
   1. Max heart rate = 220 - age = _____ (e.g., 220 - 50 = 170 b/m)
   2. Subtract resting heart rate   =   (e.g., 170 - 80 = 90 b/m)
   3. Multiply .75 (75% intensity of workload) =_____ (e.g., .75 x 90 = 67.5 b/m)
   4. Add back your resting heart rate =_____ (e.g., 67.5 + 80 = 147.5 b/m)
   5. Target heart rate =_____

6. A beginner exercise program needs a frequency of three times per week. Write down three days of the week that you can dedicate to your fitness program.

_____

7. Anything else you wish to include here:

_____

_____

_____

_____

_____

Talk to a doctor before starting any exercise routine...

[EXERCISE 3.4]

Stress-Related Eating Behaviors

Please read the following statements and circle the appropriate answer. Then tally the total to determine your score from the key below.

		4 = Always	3 = Often	2 = Sometimes	1 = Rarely				0 = Never
1.	I tend to skip breakfast on a regular basis.				4	3	2	1	0
2.	On average, two or three meals are prepared outside the home each day.				4	3	2	1	0
3.	I drink more than one cup of coffee or tea a day.				4	3	2	1	0
4.	I tend to drink more than one soda/pop per day.				4	3	2	1	0
5.	I commonly snack between meals.				4	3	2	1	0
6.	When in a hurry, I usually eat at fast food places.				4	3	2	1	0
7.	I tend to snack while watching television.				4	3	2	1	0
8.	I tend to put salt on my food before tasting it.				4	3	2	1	0
9.	I drink fewer than eight glasses of water a day.				4	3	2	1	0
10.	I tend to satisfy my sweet tooth daily.				4	3	2	1	0
11.	When preparing meals at home, I usually don't cook from scratch.				4	3	2	1	0
12.	Honestly, my eating habits lean toward fast, junk, processed foods.				4	3	2	1	0
13.	I eat fewer than 4 to 5 servings of fresh vegetables per day.				4	3	2	1	0
14.	I drink at least one glass of wine, beer, or alcohol a day.				4	3	2	1	0
15.	My meals are eaten sporadically throughout the day rather than at regularly scheduled times.				4	3	2	1	0
16.	I don't usually cook with fresh herbs and spices.				4	3	2	1	0
17.	I usually don't make a habit of eating organic fruits and veggies.				4	3	2	1	0
18.	My biggest meal of the day is usually eaten after 7:00 p.m.				4	3	2	1	0
19.	For the most part, my vitamins and minerals come from the foods I eat.				4	3	2	1	0
20.	Artificial sweeteners are in many of the foods I eat.				4	3	2	1	0

TOTALS ❭

TOTAL SCORE ❭

SCORE

A score of more than 20 points indicates that your eating behaviors are not conducive to reducing stress. A score of more than 30 suggests that your eating habits may seriously compromise the integrity of your immune system.

[EXERCISE 3.5]

The Rainbow Diet

Food color is more important than just having a nice presentation on your dinner plate. Each color holds a specific vibration in the spectrum of light. When this is combined with the nutrient value of food, it can help to enhance the health of the physical body. In the science of subtle energies, each of the body's primary chakras is associated with a specific color (see chart below). It is thought that by eating fruits and vegetables associated with the color of various chakras that this provides healthy energy to that specific region. For example, women with urinary tract infections (root chakra) are encouraged to drink cranberry juice (red). Diabetics with macular problems are encouraged to eat blueberries and take the herb bilberry (blue). Moreover, recent research suggests that the active ingredients in fruits and vegetables that give them their color are called bioflavonoids, and these are now thought to help prevent cancer. Regardless of Eastern philosophies or Western science, the bottom line is to eat a good variety of fruits and vegetables. The following list identifies the seven chakras, their respective body regions, and the color associated with each chakra/region. List five fruits, veggies, or herbs for each color.

Chakra	Body Region	Color	Food Choices
1. Crown	Pineal	Purple	_____
2. Brow	Pituitary	Indigo	_____
3. Throat	Thymus	Aqua-blue	_____
4. Heart	Heart	Green	_____
5. Solar Plexus	Adrenals	Yellow	_____
6. Navel	Spleen	Orange	_____
7. Root	Gonads	Red	_____

Additional Thoughts: _____

_____

_____

_____

_____

_____

_____

[EXERCISE 3.6]

Self-Assessment: Poor Sleep Habits Questionnaire

Please take a moment to answer these questions based on your typical behavior. If you feel your sleep quality is compromised, consider that one or more of these factors may contribute to patterns of insomnia by affecting your physiology, circadian rhythms, or emotional thought processing. Although there is no key to determine your degree of insomnia, each question is based on specific factors associated with either a good night's sleep or the lack of it. Use each question to help you fine-tune your sleep hygiene.

1.	Do you go to bed at about the same time every night?	YES	NO
2.	Does it take you more than 30 minutes to fall asleep once in bed?	YES	NO
3.	Do you wake up at about the same time every day?	YES	NO
4.	Do you drink coffee, tea, or caffeinated soda after 6 p.m.?	YES	NO
5.	Do you watch television from your bed?	YES	NO
6.	Do you perform cardiovascular exercise 3 to 5 times per week?	YES	NO
7.	Do you use your bed as your office (e.g., homework, balance checkbook, write letters, etc.)?	YES	NO
8.	Do you take a hot shower or bath before you go to sleep?	YES	NO
9.	Do you have one or more drinks of alcohol before bedtime?	YES	NO
10.	Are you engaged in intense mental activity before bed (e.g., term papers, exams, projects, reports, finances, taxes)?	YES	NO
11.	Is your bedroom typically warm or even hot before you go to bed?	YES	NO
12.	Does your sleep partner snore, become restless, etc. in the night?	YES	NO
13.	Is the size and comfort level of your bed satisfactory?	YES	NO
14.	Do you suffer from chronic pain while lying down?	YES	NO
15.	Is your sleep environment compromised by noise, light or pets?	YES	NO
16.	Do you frequently take naps during the course of a day?	YES	NO
17.	Do you take medications (e.g., decongestants, steroids, anti-hypertensives, asthma medications, or medications for depression)?	YES	NO
18.	Do you tend to suffer from depression?	YES	NO
19.	Do you eat a large heavy meal right before you go to bed?	YES	NO
20.	Do you use a cell phone regularly, particularly in the evening?	YES	NO

[EXERCISE 3.7]

Your Circadian Rhythms

Your body runs on a 24-hour clock, based on the earth spinning on its axis around the sun. Research shows that people who keep to a regular schedule tend to be healthier (less colds, flus, etc.) than those whose lifestyle behaviors tend to be more erratic. In this exercise you are asked to monitor your lifestyle behaviors based on the time of day that these occur for a full week's time.

Week of _____

CIRCADIAN RHYTHMS	SUN	MON	TUE	WED	THUR	FRI	SAT
Time you awake each morning							
Time you go to bed							
Time you fall asleep							
Time that you eat breakfast							
Time that you eat lunch							
Time that you eat dinner							
Times that you snack							
Time of bowel movements							
Time that you exercise							
Time that you have sex							
Other regular activities e.g.:							
Other regular activities e.g.:							

[CHAPTER 4]

Mental Well-Being

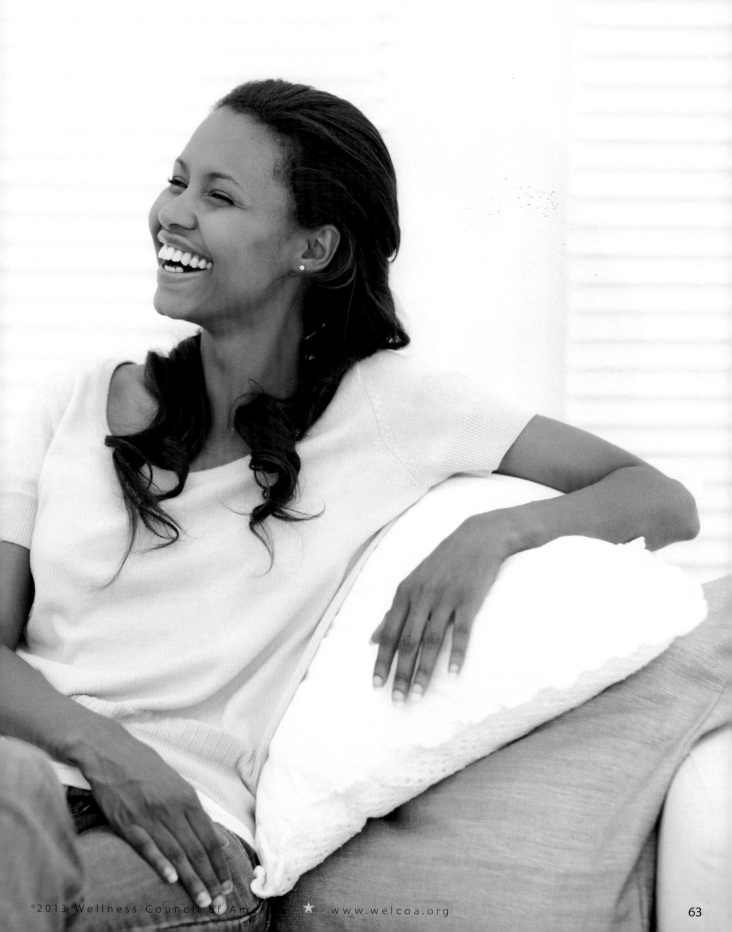

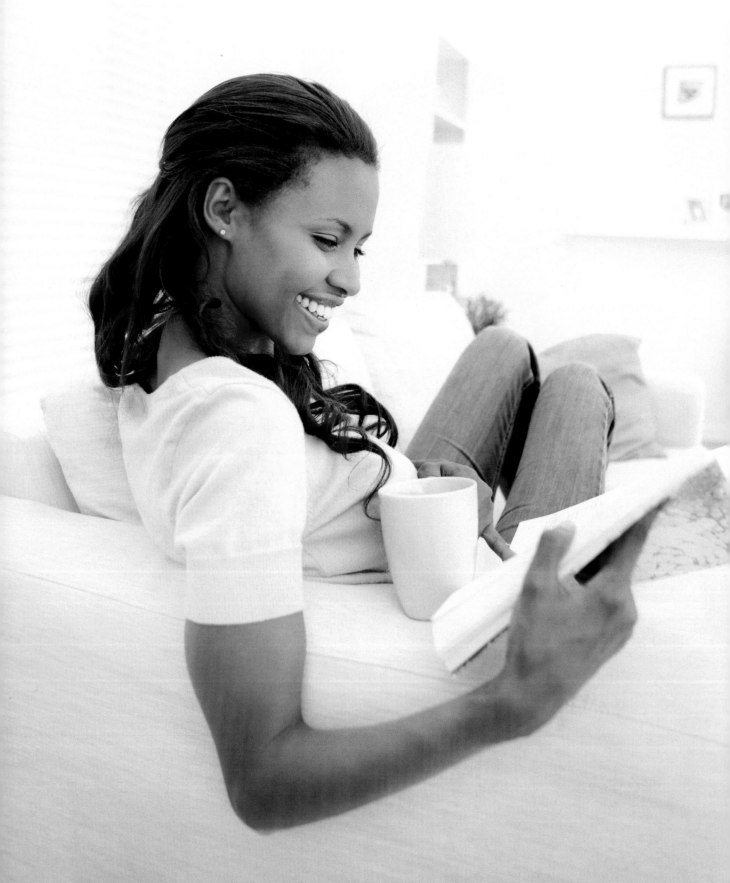

[CHAPTER 4]

Mental Well-Being

Consider this: You encounter hundreds of thousands of bits of information instantly filtered through your mind as they cascade through your five senses to the central command of your brain—on a daily basis. At first blush, this appears to be an overwhelming amount of data to comprehend, let alone process. Yet the average person does it with great ease. This estimate of sensory stimulation far exceeds that which people, only a few decades ago, would ever experience. Welcome to the information age! Today the common complaint is TMI (too much information), perhaps you have even said this expression to yourself in frustration. It's a valid complaint. With a never-ending array of high tech gadgets our distracted minds act like unsupervised, sugar-buzzed kids in a candy store. Today our brains are both distracted and assaulted repeatedly with bits and bytes of data. How we process this amount of information is still under speculation, but as scientists examine the active brain and its thought processes with the use of functional Magnetic Resonance Imaging (fMRI), we are inching toward a great comprehension of the brain (neurons and neurochemicals), the mind (consciousness) and various aspects of mental well-being. Welcome to a brave new world of consciousness. Knowledge may be power, but wisdom is enlightening.

> " Knowledge may be power, but wisdom is enlightening. "

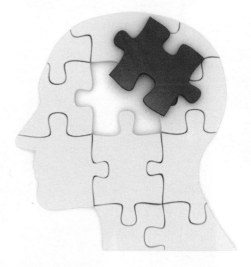

> Research reveals that indeed, the mind is amazing, but the mind needs focused discipline to do a good job.

The mind/brain is like a compact super computer. It is so amazing, with millions upon millions of neural connections, and we may only know a fraction of its dynamics. A great mind effortlessly gathers, processes, recalls and communicates information (sometimes in nano-seconds)—and that is the definition of mental well-being: the ability to gather, process, recall and communicate information. At our best, each of these abilities is a marvel, yet even the mind, and more so the brain, has its limits. As such, we need to do our best to cultivate a balance between sensory stimulation and mental tranquility. Indeed, the mind craves stimulation, yet the mind needs its share of quite time as well. Mental well-being is nothing less than a balance of mental stimulation and mental relaxation. Once achieved, its potential is nothing less than astonishing.

The Myth Of Multi-Tasking

While it may seem like doing two things at once (e.g., texting and cooking dinner) saves time (and perhaps even appears to be well-organized), the bottom line is that we end up doing a sloppy job with both tasks. No better example illustrates this point than texting and driving. Research reveals that indeed, the mind is amazing, but the mind needs focused discipline to do a good job. Productive focusing skills are a rare commodity these days (note the abundance of people with some level of Attention Deficit Disorder). Studies show that not only does the quality of work productivity suffer with a distracted mind, but mistakes are often made, resulting in greater time inefficiency. Sadly, we live in a fast-paced world of immediate gratification where the practice of multi-tasking is common. However, the verdict is in: Don't multi-task. Stay focused on one thing at a time until it's done, and then move on to the next. It's that simple.

Brain Fog, Sensory Overload And Neuroplasticity

As great as the mind/brain is, there are limits to its abilities. Scientists are now learning that too much sensory stimulation begins to create neural pathways (and chemical processes that use these neural pathways) to assimilate this wealth of information, yet in the process it also creates stress in the brain. This stress is now known to shrink brain tissue. The bottom line is that too much mental stimulation becomes sensory overload, compromising our mental well-being. Without giving the mind a chance to rest (and process this information) thinking processes become clouded, or what is now called brain fog. And while it was once thought that our brain cells were finite (determined at birth) we now know that brain cells and their associated neural pathways are being created all the time as a result of our exposure to the sensory stimulation we encounter. Neuroscientists refer to this as neuroplasticity. The good news is that neuroplasticity is also created through the use of other cognitive skills like meditation; a skilled activity that promotes a tranquil mind and the brain that houses it.

Left Brain-Right Brain Thinking

Years ago it was discovered that we really don't have one brain. Rather, we have two brains connected together with an amazing set of neural pathways called the corpus callosum. Each half of the brain (left and right hemispheres) contains a unique set of thinking skills and specific ways to perceive the world. The left side of the brain is quite adept at logic, reasoning, verbal skills, facts and figures, and judgment as well as several other skills used in the flight or fight response. Conversely, the right brain holds the acumen of intuition, imagination, global thinking and skills associated with artistic talent and relaxation. Together these two halves form a most remarkable and powerful alliance of cognition. It has been noted, however, that the American culture is left-brain dominant, meaning that we tend to favor the left-brain cognitive skills and ignore the other half, leaving one at a deficit of consciousness. Right-brain thinking skills are crucial for optimal mental well-being.

The Power Of Two Minds

For eons, the mind, not to mention the processes of conscious thought, has always seemed to be quite abstract and hard to describe accurately. In such cases we tend to use metaphors to illustrate the indescribable. For example, the mind is often compared to an iceberg; the conscious mind is that part of the iceberg above the water, whereas the unconscious mind is that which is below the water. The conscious mind is alert during the waking hours, yet it shuts down completely during sleep. The unconscious mind never stops working in an effort to help the conscious mind navigate the world. Mental well-being is more than just accessing both hemispheres of the brain. It is also combining forces of the conscious and unconscious minds. Interestingly enough, the unconscious mind has a different set of language skills than the conscious mind. The unconscious mind communicates in the expression of symbols, metaphors, stories, colors and dream images. The unconscious mind has a lot to say and much to offer in terms of deep-seated wisdom. Mental well-being is greatly (and often unknowingly) compromised, however, when the conscious mind, unable to interpret these messages, ignores the wisdom conveyed through this language. Since the early days of psychology with Sigmund Freud and Carl Jung leading the way, we now know that the unconscious mind governs behavior. When we take the time to bridge the understanding of these two minds, we are better equipped to make positive behavior changes that last. Without the help of the unconscious mind, these efforts for positive change are fruitless.

> Mental well-being is greatly (and often unknowingly) compromised, however, when the conscious mind, unable to interpret these messages, ignores the wisdom conveyed through this language.

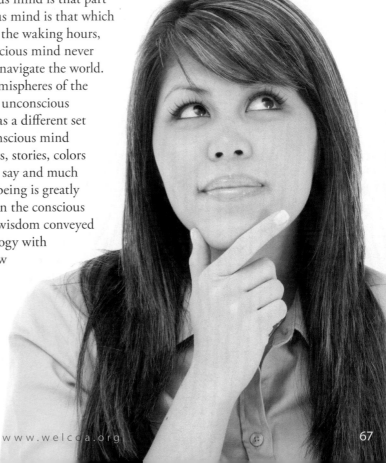

> " Perhaps most interesting is the research that reveals people who have an optimistic outlook on various aspects of life tend to have an enhanced immune system. "

Ego As Bodyguard, Not CEO

To speak of mental well-being without mentioning the ego would be a gross injustice to both topics. Your ego is your bodyguard (it is what sets off the alarm for the fight or flight response to ensure physical survival). You need your ego! But the ego is only supposed to be your bodyguard, nothing more. When it ascends to the level of CEO it usually spells trouble. It has been suggested that an excess of left-brain thinking gives the ego free rein to call the shots in terms of conscious thought. The good life requires that one keeps the ego in check on a regular basis.

The Power Of Positive Thinking

Ask any Olympic athlete if they believe in the power of positive thinking and they will grin. At that level of competition where physical ability is uniform among competitors, it's one's attitude that determines the winner. Many cancer survivors will say the same thing. There is no room for negativity in achieving greatness or health for that matter. Negative thoughts are self-defeating. The power of positive thinking has been studied for decades and made popular with the likes of Norman Vincent Peale and Deepak Chopra. Perhaps most interesting is the research that reveals people who have an optimistic outlook on various aspects of life tend to have an enhanced immune system. Furthermore, consider the dynamics of the conscious and unconscious minds. Both need to be on board for positive thinking to be effective (e.g., words and phrases for conscious thought and symbolic images for the unconscious mind).

Think of your thoughts as energy. Positive energy expands. Negative energy contracts. This is not to say we should wear rose-colored glasses all the time (remember, every emotional thought needs time to be recognized and processed), yet in a world filled with fear-mongering and negativity, positive thinking becomes an essential asset in achieving the good life. Is your glass half full or half empty? It all comes down to perspective and attitude. Please consider using Exercise 4.1 (Reframing) as a means to help you find balance with your thoughts.

Creativity And The Creative Solving Process

Creativity is one of the attributes that separates humans from all other life forms on the planet. Birds may build nests in trees, but humans have created the Taj Mahal, Buckingham Palace, the Acropolis and the Pyramids of Giza. Beavers may create damns in rivers, but humans can create cell phones, the space shuttle and the Mona Lisa. If you think about it, every great invention began as an idea in someone's head. Creativity isn't a gift for a chosen few; it's a birthright for everyone.

Einstein once said that logic will get you from A to B, but imagination will get you everywhere. He was right. Those who have studied creativity and the creative process have come to the realization that it's not simply a right-brain function, it's a whole brain function! Ideas may begin with one's imagination, but a great idea that never sees the light of day isn't very creative. There has to be an end product. The left-brain skills of judgment and organization are necessary to make a good idea come to fruition. Exercise 4.2 outlines the steps of the creative process through the work of creativity consultant and author, Roger von Oech.

Researchers in the field of psychology have noted that people who exercise their sense of creativity are quite simply happy people. They revel in the creative process. Researchers have also realized that when people employ their creative abilities to problem solve they feel a sense of empowerment. Empowerment is another word for mental well-being. Do you need a nudge with your sense of creativity? Try completing exercise 4.3, *My Creativity Project*. See where this takes you. Remember, Rome wasn't built in a day. Finally, is there a problem that you need to solve? Let exercise 4.4 walk you through the steps of the creative problem solving process.

Meditation: It's Not What You Think

Mark describes his thought process as "monkey-mind," a term he picked up years ago while in India on a business trip. Monkey mind is a common eastern expression that describes a mind running all over the place; a mind that is never still. When he got home Mark changed the term to "squirrel mind" because as he said, there are no monkeys in New York but we have plenty of squirrels! No matter what it's called, the end result is the same; a flurry of frantic distracting thoughts that cascade through the nervous system. It wasn't squirrel mind that got Mark interested in meditation; it was a high blood pressure reading before dental surgery. Faced with the reality of being on prescribed meds, Mark took the initiative to change some behaviors. The goal was to get rid of squirrel mind, not to mention better systolic and diastolic readings. At first it was hard, he admitted. Sitting still for five minutes seemed like an eternity. But he stuck with it. "I begin with a pad of paper and pen by my side and I focus on my breathing. With each distracting thought, I write down whatever pops up. Writing it down gets it out of my head. I now meditate for 30 minutes each morning before I head to work. It's amazing what a simple breathing exercise can do for your health. I can now see in others the behaviors I used to have and shake my head in disbelief. How can people live like this? I am happy to say I don't have squirrel mind anymore. I don't have hypertension anymore, either."

> Researchers in the field of psychology have noted that people who exercise their sense of creativity are quite simply happy people.

> Meditation is a time-tested method that calms the mind so you can gain a better sense of focus and concentration (two aspects lacking in today's rapidly paced lifestyles).

What is the antidote to sensory overload? The answer is meditation. Meditation is a time-tested method that calms the mind so you can gain a better sense of focus and concentration (two aspects lacking in today's rapidly paced lifestyles). Meditation goes by several names including mindfulness, centering, the relaxation response and mental training (a term used by Olympic athletes to increase their concentration skills for better performance).

The purpose of meditation is to increase concentration and awareness, nothing more. A secondary goal is to domesticate the ego by putting it back in its place as bodyguard. A practice of meditation involves sitting quietly and focusing on your breathing. By limiting (focusing) your stream of thoughts to one thing (e.g., your breathing), you clear out the ego chitter-chatter with non-essential (often fear-based) thoughts. Meditation brings you to the present moment, and this is one of its greatest benefits.

Research reveals that the benefits of a regular meditation practice are amazing, and not just for the mind, but the body and spirit as well. Here is a short list:

> ❯ Increased concentration (attention) skills
> ❯ Increased creativity
> ❯ Increased quality of sleep
> ❯ Increased immune system function
> ❯ Decreased resting blood pressure
> ❯ Decreased resting heart rate
> ❯ Decreased muscle tension

There are thousands of ways to meditate and often people use guided mental imagery as a way to introduce themselves to this routine. Exercise 4.5 includes two meditation scripts to read through (or have someone read to you) while you relax. As with all types of mental imagery, remember to engage the five senses and take what aspects of the meditation script you like and disregard the rest.

The Art Of Calm

Today there is a growing emphasis on personal health and wellness at the worksite and the effects that stress plays on disease and illness. As the pace of life increases it becomes imperative to take time to relax. Keeping aware of the fact that there is no separation between the mind and body, a stressed mind results in a stressed body. Yes, the mind can become overwhelmed with sensory stimulation (as evidenced by the new social disease called screen addiction). But it's also true that we can take in relaxing stimulation through the five senses (the portals of the nervous system) to calm both the mind and body.

What are some of the best ways to relax? To be honest, there are hundreds of ways, but they all fall into one of five categories: Sight, sound, taste, touch and smell. The premise of the art of calm invites us to use the five senses to gain a sense of balance. Examples include but are not limited to: listening to calm relaxing music, inhaling the scent of lavender or balsam fir, enjoying the taste of juicy watermelon on a hot afternoon, or getting a soothing muscle massage. How do you find joy in life? Perhaps it's by engaging one or more of the five senses with some pleasing sensory stimulus. Exercise 4.6 asks you to make a list of ways to relax through the five senses.

> " The premise of the art of calm invites us to use the five senses to gain a sense of balance. "

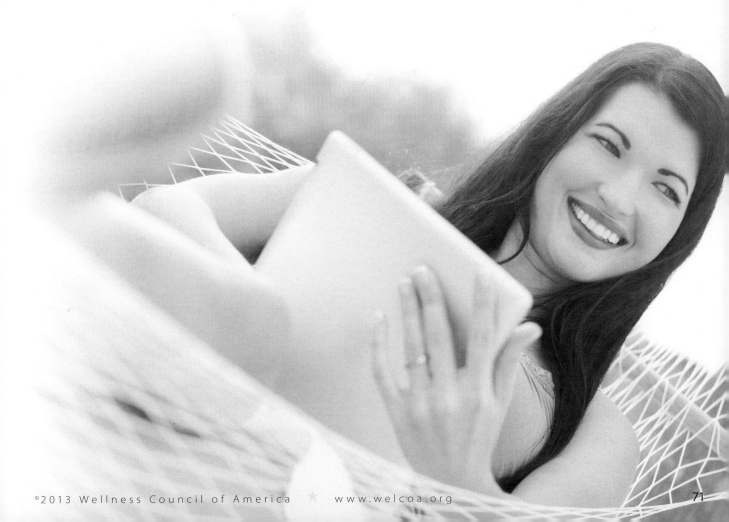

[EXERCISE 4.1]

Reframing: Seeing A Bigger, Clearer Perspective

Anger and fear-based thoughts that arise from encountering a stressful situation can narrow our focus of the bigger picture. Although the initial aspects of dealing with these situations involves some degree of grieving, the secret to coping with stress is to change the threatening perception to a non-threatening perception. This worksheet invites you to identify three stressors and, if necessary, draft a new "reframed" positive perspective (not a rationalization) that allows you to get out of the rut of a myopic view and start moving on with your life.

1. Situation: _____

_____

Reframed Perspective _____

_____

2. Situation: _____

_____

Reframed Perspective _____

_____

3. Situation: _____

_____

Reframed Perspective _____

_____

[EXERCISE 4.2]

The Roles Of Creativity

Creativity consultant Roger von Oech is right when he states that many hats are worn in the creative process! Reviewing these four specific roles (and the specific order they are in), please take some time to examine how you can integrate these creative aspects into your repertoire of cognitive skills. If you are like most people, you tend to see yourself as wearing only one of these hats, rather than all four. This is OK when projects or problems require a team effort. For now, let's assume that you can wear all four hats and wear them well.

I. The Explorer: **To help you think outside the box, make a list of five new places you can explore to find new ideas for any creative project. Next, make a list of five new resources to explore for any creative project.**

1. _____
2. _____
3. _____
4. _____
5. _____

II. The Artist: **Inside each and every one of us is an artist begging to play. Make a list of five new ways to engage in the art of play!**

1. _____
2. _____
3. _____
4. _____
5. _____

III. The Judge: **How good are your judgment skills? Are they too good? Are you the kind of person who judges first and asks questions later?**

_____
_____
_____
_____

IV. The Warrior: **The warrior is the "leg man" in the creative process. A great idea without someone to market it and implement it is not really a great idea. How good are your warrior skills? What can you do to improve them?**

_____
_____
_____
_____

[EXERCISE 4.3]

My Creativity Project

This exercise is geared to help inspire you to take some initiative in starting and completing a project that requires some creative license. Initially, this assignment was developed for a holistic health class to fully engage students in the creative process. Many people found this project to be the ticket to a new job. The purpose of this exercise is to challenge you to extend your creative talents to your highest limits. This project involves three aspects:

Part I: First, play the role of the explorer, artist, judge and warrior respectively, to come up with a very creative idea and then bring it to reality. If you wish, you can use the template in *The Roles of Creativity* exercise again for this exercise.

Part II: Next, describe your experience: what you did (describe your experience in each of the four stages of creativity) and how you accomplished it.

Part III: Finally, explain what you learned from this experience.

The area and magnitude of creativity is entirely up to you. It is suggested, however, that you pick an area that is somewhat familiar (in other words, don't try to build the Brooklyn Bridge if you have never even played with Legos), but not one in which you have a five-star command. Challenge yourself! Select a project which can range anywhere from art, poetry, cooking, composing, photography, designing fashions, writing a screenplay, choreographing a dance—anything! Start with an interest, passion, or a craving desire. Build from this a dream. Consult your intuition and then come up with a finished product. Remember that the creative process cannot be rushed or demanded. This assignment will take some time, so plan accordingly.

Additional Tips

Make the project manageable, but challenging. For example, simply putting a new message on your answering machine is not the best way to go. Make the project a quality job and one in which you will be proud.

The following are examples from previous students and workshop participants:

> ❯ Producing a music video
> ❯ Recording/producing a musical CD
> ❯ Writing a family/neighborhood cookbook
> ❯ Planning a vacation around the world
> ❯ Producing a multi-media presentation
> ❯ Designing/planting a rose garden
> ❯ Creating a holistic cancer treatment plan
> ❯ Writing a nonfiction book proposal

My Creativity Project: _____

_____

_____

_____

How I Did It: _____

_____

_____

_____

_____

_____

_____

_____

What I Learned: _____

_____

_____

_____

_____

_____

_____

[EXERCISE 4.4]

Creative Problem Solving

There are many good ways to solve a problem! All you need to do is spend some time working at it from different directions until a number of creative, viable solutions surface, and then choose the best one. The following is a time-tested strategic plan for creatively solving problems.

The Problem: _____

_____

_____

_____

_____

I. Define/Describe The Problem (Please be as specific as you can):

_____

_____

_____

_____

_____

II. Generating Great Ideas (Come up with at least four viable ideas and one zany one to bring out the play factor):

1. _____

2. _____

3. _____

4. _____

(x). _____

III. Idea Selection & Refinement (Pick the best idea from above and explain why you think this is the best idea):

_____

_____

_____

_____

_____

IV. Idea Implementation (Explain how you will put this idea into action. Make a brief outline—four specific points of your action plan to make this happen):

_____

_____

_____

_____

_____

V. Evaluation & Analysis Of Your Action Plan (How did the idea work? What are some ways to improve on this idea should you decide to use it again?)

_____

_____

_____

_____

_____

[EXERCISE 4.5]

Guided Mental Imagery Meditation:

Solitude Of A Mountain Lake

Imagery Script: Imagine yourself walking alone in the early morning, along a path of a primeval forest, through a gauntlet of towering pine trees. Each step you take is softly cushioned by a bed of golden-brown needles. Quietness consumes these surroundings and then is broken by the melody of a songbird. As you stroll along at a leisurely pace, you focus on the sweet, clean scent of the pines and evergreens, the coolness of the air, the warmth of the sun as it peeks through the trees, and the gentle breeze as it passes through the boughs of the pines and whispers past your ears.

Off in the distance, you hear the rush of water cascading over weathered rocks, babbling as it moves along. Yards ahead, a chipmunk perches on an old decaying birch stump along the side of the path, frozen momentarily to determine its next direction, then in the blink of an eye, it disappears under the ground cover and all is silent again. As you continue to walk along this path, you see a clearing up ahead, and you notice your pace picks up just a little to see what is up ahead. First boulders appear ahead, then behind them, a deep blue mountain lake emerges from beyond the rocks. You climb up on a boulder to secure a better view, and you find a comfortable spot carved out of the weathered stone to sit and quietly observe all the elements around you.

The shore of the lake is surrounded by a carpet of tall green grass and guarded by a host of trees: spruce, evergreen, pine, aspen, and birch. On top of one of the spruce trees, an eagle leaves his perch and spreads his wings to catch the remains of a thermal current, and gracefully glides over the lake. On the far side of the lake, off in the distance, dwarfing the tree line, is a rugged stone face mountain. The first snows of autumn have dusted the fissures and crevasses adding contrast to the rock's features. The color of the snow matches the one or two puffy white clouds and morning crescent moon that interrupt an otherwise cloudless day. A slight warm breeze begins to caress your cheeks and the backs of your hands as you direct your attention to the surface of the mountain lake.

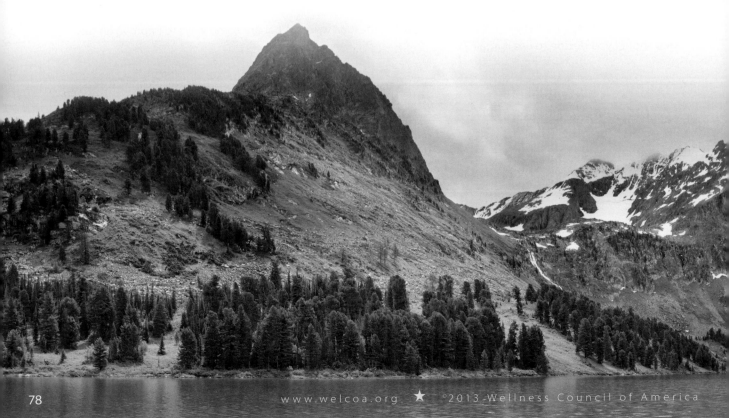

The slight breeze sends tiny ripples across the surface of the lake. As you look at the water's surface, you realize that this body of water, this mountain lake, is just like your body, somewhat calm, yet yearning to be completely relaxed, completely calm. Focus your attention on the surface of the water. These ripples that you observe represent or symbolize any tensions, frustrations or wandering thoughts that keep you from being completely relaxed. As you look at the surface of this mountain lake, slowly allow the ripples to dissipate, fade away and disappear. To enhance this process take a very slow deep breath and feel the relaxation this brings to your body as you exhale. And as you exhale, slowly allow the ripples to fade away giving way to a calm surface of water. As you continue to focus on this image, you see the surface of the lake becoming more and more calm, in fact very placid, reflecting all that surrounds it.

As you focus on this image and realize that this body of water is like your body, take note of how relaxed you feel as you see the surface of the lake remain perfectly still, reflecting all that is around it. The water's surface reflects a mirror image of the green grass, the trees, the mountain face, even the clouds and crescent moon. Your body is as relaxed as this body of water, this mountain lake. Try to lock in this feeling of calmness and etch this feeling into your memory bank so that you can call it up to your conscious mind when you get stressed or frustrated. Remember this image so that you can recall the serenity of this image that you have created to promote a deep sense of relaxation, and feel your body relax just by thinking of the solitude of this mountain lake.

Now, slowly allow this image to fade from your mind's eye, but retain the sense of tranquility it inspired. Make yourself aware of your surroundings; the room, the building, the time of day, and perhaps what you will do after this relaxation session. Although you feel relaxed, you don't feel tired. You feel rested and rejuvenated. Begin to make yourself aware of your body. Stretch your arms and shoulders and wiggle your fingers and toes. When you feel ready, open your eyes to a soft gaze in front, and as you do, retain this sense of calm comfort all throughout your mind, body and spirit all day long.

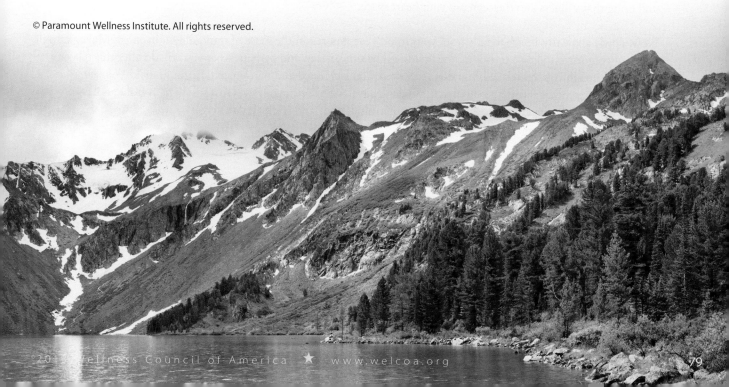

Guided Mental Imagery Meditation (continued)

Gentle Falling Snow

Imagery Script: Picture this: You are sitting by a large picture window in a warm log cabin on a brisk winter's day. You have the entire place to yourself and the solitude feels invigorating. There is a log fire in the wood stove radiating abundant heat. Both the sounds of crackling wood and the scent of pine arouses your senses and for a moment, you close your eyes and take a slow deep breath; a sigh that refreshes. As you exhale, you feel a wonderful sense of relaxation permeate your entire body from head to toe and it feels great. Consciously, you take another slow deep breath in through your nose. As you exhale through your mouth, you become aware of the glorious stillness that surrounds you in this cabin.

From where you are seated, look out the window and as you do, you see falling snow. Snow that falls gently to the ground in large flakes. Everything outside is covered in white fluffy snow; the ground, the pine trees, the aspens, in fact all the trees for as far as you can see are covered in snow. As you look closely at the snowflakes descending from on high toward the ground, you sense a calmness both indoors and outdoors. Other than snow falling, everything is still. Everything is quiet. This stillness you observe is a reflection of the tranquility you feel within yourself.

This stillness is so inviting that you slowly move off the couch and stand up. As you walk toward the cabin door, you put on your warm winter coat, hat and gloves. Then, slowly you open the door and simply stand in the doorframe to observe the endless dance of millions of snowflakes floating gently, almost in slow motion, from the sky down to the snow covered ground.

Listen closely. What do you hear? The sound of snowflakes is so soft, so gentle the sound is barely audible. If you listen very carefully, you will hear the barely audible sounds of falling snow. Your ability to focus on this sound, to the exclusion of all other thoughts, sets your mind at ease, like a broom that gently sweeps the floor of any remnants needed to be cleaned. The snow-covered ground is a symbol of your mind—clean, clear and still. Take a slow deep breath of this clean, fresh air and feel a deeper sense of calmness all throughout your entire body.

As you step back inside and close the door, you kick off your shoes, take off this jacket, hat and gloves and return to the couch by the picture window. As you close your eyes to focus on the sounds of stillness; take one final slow deep breath and bring that stillness into the center of your heart space.

Now, slowly allow this image to fade from your mind's eye, but retain the sense of tranquility it inspired. Make yourself aware of your surroundings; the room, the building, the time of day, and perhaps what you will do after this relaxation session. Although you feel relaxed, you don't feel tired. You feel rested and rejuvenated. Begin to make yourself aware of your body. Stretch your arms and shoulders. When you feel ready, open your eyes to a soft gaze in front and as you do retain this sense of calm comfort all throughout your mind, body and spirit all day long.

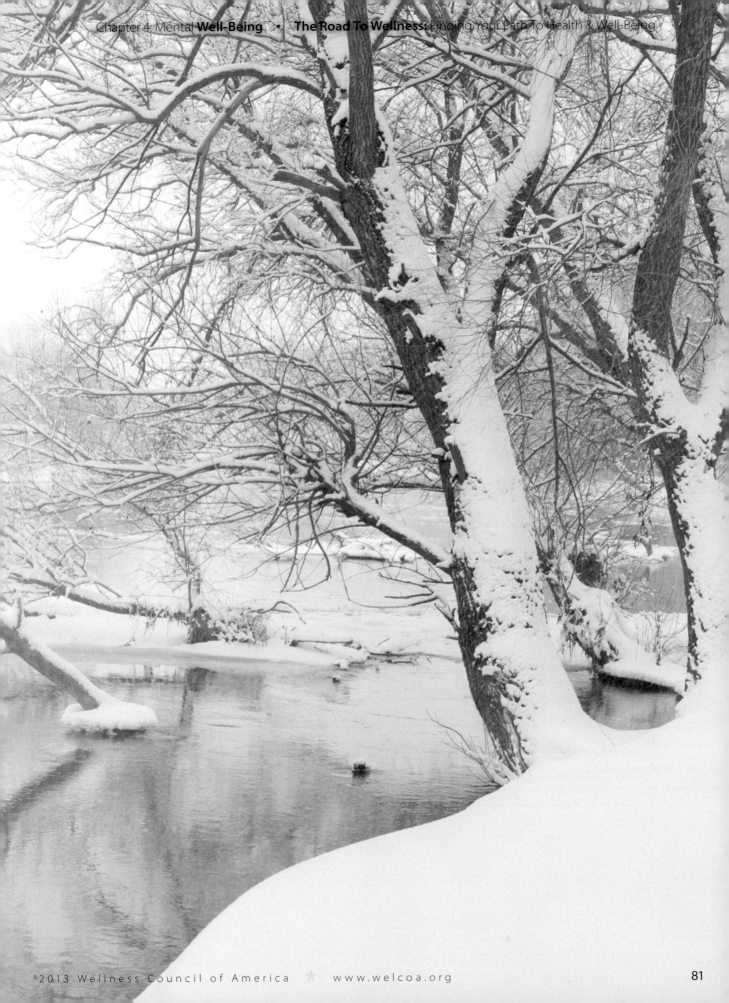

[EXERCISE 4.6]

The Art Of Calm: Relaxation Through The Five Senses

Please list 10 ideas for mind-body relaxation for each of the five senses. Note that a sixth category, the divine sense, was added for any ideas that might be a combination of these or perhaps something beyond the five senses (e.g., watching a child being born). Describe each in a few words to a sentence. Be as specific as possible, and be creative! Once you have created this list, post it somewhere where you can see it regularly in the hopes that you begin to participate in more of these art of calm experiences.

The Sense Of Sight

1. _____ 6. _____
2. _____ 7. _____
3. _____ 8. _____
4. _____ 9. _____
5. _____ 10. _____

The Sense Of Taste

1. _____ 6. _____
2. _____ 7. _____
3. _____ 8. _____
4. _____ 9. _____
5. _____ 10. _____

The Sense Of Sound

1. _____ 6. _____
2. _____ 7. _____
3. _____ 8. _____
4. _____ 9. _____
5. _____ 10. _____

The Sense Of Touch

1. _____
2. _____
3. _____
4. _____
5. _____

6. _____
7. _____
8. _____
9. _____
10. _____

The Sense Of Smell

1. _____
2. _____
3. _____
4. _____
5. _____

6. _____
7. _____
8. _____
9. _____
10. _____

The "Divine" Sense

1. _____
2. _____
3. _____
4. _____
5. _____

6. _____
7. _____
8. _____
9. _____
10. _____

[CHAPTER 5]

Emotional Well-Being

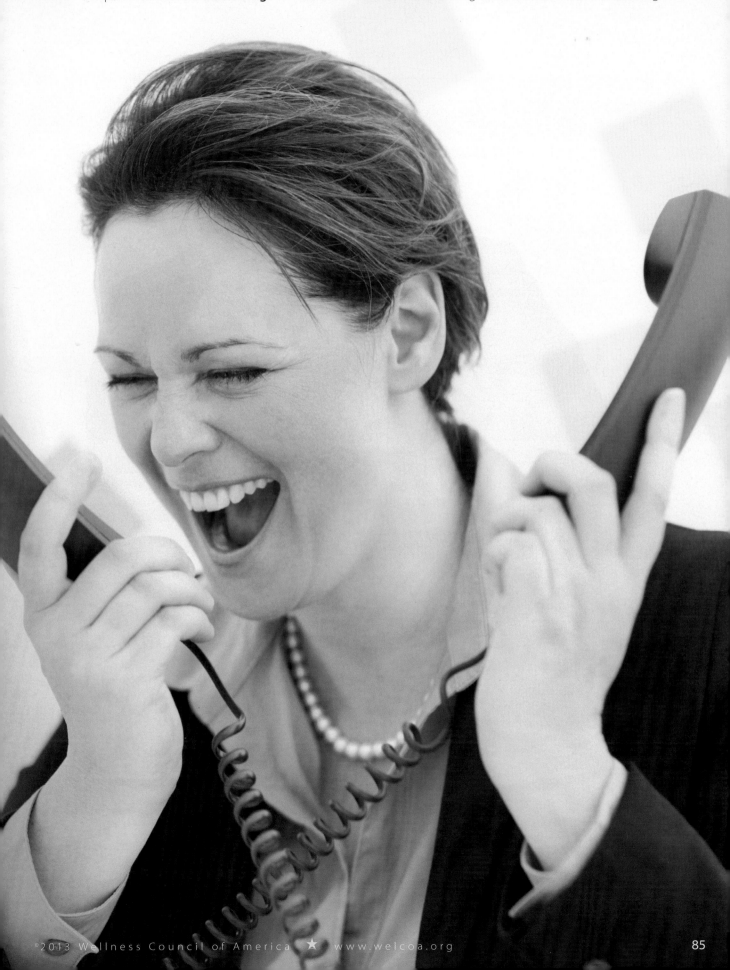

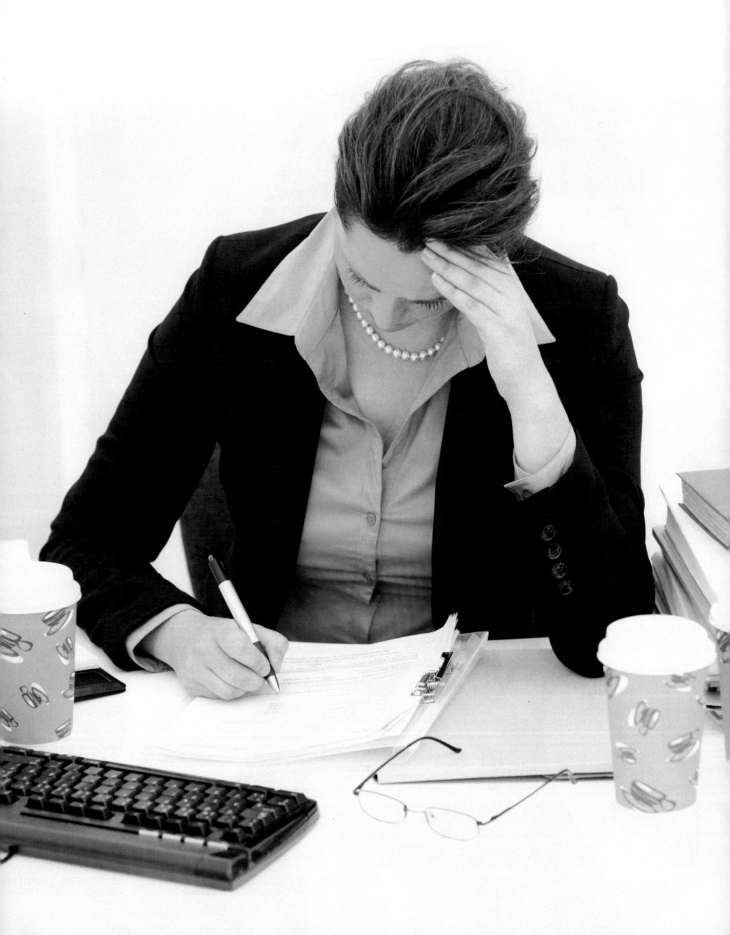

[CHAPTER 5]

Emotional Well-Being

"To laugh often and love much" is the beginning of a famous quote by Ralph Waldo Emerson commonly found floating around the Internet, Facebook and Pinterest these days. But what you're more likely to find floating around office cubicles and water coolers is a cloud of stress, masking itself as complaints, whining, or a multitude of daily frustrations. There is no shortage of these stressed-based emotions (also known as emotional baggage) in modern America. Given the amount of stress in our culture today, it's fair to say that strong emotional well-being is a rare commodity. Quite likely, the lack of emotional well-being is tied to many health-related problems associated with physical well-being. In the paradigm of holistic wellness, there is no separation between our emotions and our physical body, which is all the more reason why emotional well-being is so important to your health.

It's normal (and healthy) to feel anxious now and then, even frustrated at times. However, it's neither normal, nor healthy, to be constantly anxious or angry. As we all know, people *do* get stuck in a rut of emotions, from holding grudges to always making mountains out of molehills. All the while, the pursuit of happiness becomes ever elusive. As the expression goes, "Fear and anger rob people of the pleasure of the present moment's joy and happiness." How true! Ironically, there is an illusion of control with

> **Fear and anger rob people of the pleasure of the present moment's joy and happiness.**

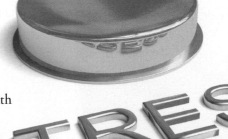

> Anger and fear are two emotions that have one purpose: to save your life in the event of physical danger.

unresolved feelings of anger and fear; you may feel like you are controlling others (or yourself), but in reality, you are giving your personal power away. The end result is to lead a life spinning around in a whirlpool of negativity. Stated differently, attitude is the paintbrush we choose to color the world.

Emotional well-being is the ability to feel and express the entire range of human emotions (from anger to love), and control them, not be controlled by them. This may sound like a tall order to fill, but healthy emotional well-being is not impossible. It does take a bit of effort to not let your feelings run wild. To state the obvious: Living in a constant state of anxiety or frustration is the antithesis of the good life.

An Abundance Of Anger And Fear

When you first meet Tom you would never know he has unresolved anger issues (that go back many years). Tom is the kind of guy who always has a smile on his face, yet there is often a deep undercurrent of nervous laughter with each smile. "Don't rock the boat" is one of his familiar expressions. He wears a night guard for his teeth when he sleeps because he suffers from temporomandibular joint dysfunction (TMJ). Tom is a classic case of a *Somatizer*; someone who suppresses his/her anger. It was a survival skill he learned early on in life. As the child of two abusive alcoholic parents, he learned quickly not to draw attention to himself, in an effort to minimize physical and emotional abuse. What was a survival skill in childhood has come back to haunt him as an adult. That is until he took an anger management class. Now he is beginning to change his thoughts and behaviors in healthy ways. He has learned that anger has its place in tiny amounts. Tom still smiles a lot, but now there are no undercurrents of tension. And he no longer has to wear his night guard.

Anger and fear are two emotions that have one purpose: to save your life in the event of physical danger. Anger is the fight response. Fear is the flight response. Believe it or not, they are healthy emotions for the purpose of personal safety. For example, you would want fear to kick in (and quick) if the building you were in catches on fire. Anger comes in handy to defend yourself when your personal space is invaded. Since it doesn't take much time to escape from danger, it would stand to reason that the experience of fear or anger shouldn't last very long, perhaps only minutes or seconds. Yet, people are known to carry anxieties and frustrations (grudges) for weeks, years, even decades. There are many types of fear. Perhaps the most common of these is the fear of the unknown. Since most of us don't have good psychic abilities, common sense must prevail. When faced with the unknown, take time to gather information, learn what you can and respond, don't react. The antidote for worry is to strategically plan for the future, and let go of things you cannot control. Planning creates as sense of empowerment. Worry, an immobilizing aspect of fear, ends up depleting your personal energy.

There is a lot of anger looming in the air these days. Perhaps you have noticed. Road rage. Sports rage. Election rage. Tarmac rage. Even gas pump rage; not to mention rage in the form of elementary school and movie theater shootings. None of this is good; in fact it's extremely bad. Experts in the field of anger management have noted that when anger lasts longer than a few moments, it becomes a control issue called "mismanaged anger." These same experts have noticed that mismanaged anger reveals itself in one of four ways, each of which is unbecoming human behavior, but very common in our society.

The first style of mismanaged anger is called the *Somatizer*. The word soma means body in Latin. The *Somatizer* is someone who never gets angry. Rather than express their anger, they suppress it. By doing so, the body becomes the battlefield for the war games of the mind. Suppressed anger manifests itself in many health-related issues, from temporomandibular joint dysfunction (TMJ) and migraine headaches to a whole host of auto-immune diseases (e.g., lupus, rheumatoid arthritis and fibromyalgia). The *Exploder* is the second style of mismanaged anger. These people erupt like a volcano with their hot lava used as an expression of intimidation. Road rage is a prime example. So is swearing. The third style is called the *Self-punisher*. These people feel guilty about feeling angry (guilt is a form of anger) and then turn their guilt into an obsessive compulsive behavior such as excess eating, exercise, sleep or shopping to name a few. Self-mutilation (also known as cutting) falls in this category. The fourth style of mismanaged anger is known as the *Underhander*, whose motto is "Don't get mad, get even." Sarcasm, showing up late for meetings and withholding information are prime examples of the *Underhander's* style. Also known as passive-aggressive behavior, underhanded behavior is the most common style used at the worksite.

While we may exhibit all of these mismanaged anger styles (unless you are a *Somatizer*), typically one style rises to the top of our personality profile. Exercise 5.1, *Anger Recognition Checklist*, is a personal inventory to see if you are aware of how anger may surface in your emotional behavior. Exercise 5.2, *Mismanaged Anger Style Indicator*, is a questionnaire to help you to identify your mismanaged anger style.

> The average person tends to get angry between 15 and 20 times a day.

> Joy, happiness and bliss are also found when one exercises their funny bone to create some comic relief.

Creative Anger Management

The average person tends to get angry between 15 and 20 times a day. Each time feelings of anger surface it is the result of an unmet expectation. How do you turn mismanaged anger into creative anger management? The first step is to acknowledge one's mismanaged anger style. The next step is to fine-tune one's expectations. After this, you must learn how to either side step issues that press your anger buttons or come to terms with the issues that upset you and work to resolve them. Figure 5.1 and 5.2 illustrate poor and well-managed anger styles, respectively. Exercise 5.3 walks you through a 10-step program for healthy anger management.

Joy, Happiness And Bliss

Have you noticed a plethora of book titles and television specials these days on the topic of happiness? Everyone, it seems, is in search of the pot of gold at the end of the emotional rainbow, and for good reason; happiness feels good. Thomas Jefferson even highlighted happiness into the Declaration of Independence: Life, liberty and the pursuit of happiness. Experts in the field of positive psychology agree that much of what joy and happiness consists of is gratitude; taking time to appreciate what you have rather than wishing for what you don't have. Joy, happiness and bliss are also found when one exercises their funny bone to create some comic relief.

What brings happiness? So often we try to achieve happiness with material possessions, but this only provides a temporary fix. Happiness is an inside job. The good life is the happy life! So, what makes you happy? If your answer includes good friends, good health and good times you are basking in the light of the happiness rainbow. In words often attributed to Ben Franklin, "The Declaration of Independence only guarantees the American people the *right* to pursue happiness. You have to catch it yourself." Sometimes the path to happiness is taking stock of what you already have. Exercise 5.4, *1,000 Things Went Right Today!* invites you to count your blessings.

Comic Relief: The Healing Power Of Humor

Andrew is a software engineer for a company outside of Boston. From his emails, tweets, and Facebook postings you can tell he has one heck of a sense of humor. What you cannot tell is that Andrew is a quadriplegic. The day before his 13th birthday he suffered a severe spinal injury while playing around in his backyard swimming pool with his brother. Andrew's road to recovery was long and hard. However, he met a nurse in rehab hospital and she opened the door to humor as an essential tool for health and healing. He is forever grateful. "I cannot use my legs, and I can barely use my arms, but my funny bone is the strongest bone in my body," he says with an ear-to-ear smile. "People take themselves way too seriously today. Look at me. I have had a rough life, but I don't let it get me down. Nurturing my sense of humor has been my salvation." He adds with another smile. "Make it your salvation too!"

To laugh often is right. Laughter is definitely great medicine for the soul. In fact, you can find this stated in the Bible: A merry heart does good like medicine. (Proverbs, 17:22). Experts suggest that we need at least 15 laughs a day for our health, more if possible. These same experts suggest that laughter is not only good for emotional health, but it's also good for your physical health as well. Laughter helps decrease muscle tension, decrease resting blood pressure and increase neurochemicals to make you feel good. Your funny bone needs a workout as much as your cardiovascular system. Here are some suggestions to flex your funny bone:

1. Look for one funny thing a day. It could be a cartoon, a joke, or funny Youtube video. If you look for one funny thing a day you're very likely to find many things to make you smile and laugh. Here are some funny quotes to get you started:

"No matter how cynical you become, it's never enough to keep up."
—Lily Tomlin

"Some guy hit my fender, and I told him, 'Be fruitful and multiply,' but not in those words."
—Woody Allen

"I used to be Snow White, but I drifted."
—Mae West

"My wife was afraid of the dark... then she saw me naked and now she's afraid of the light."
—Rodney Dangerfield

"Depression... is anger without the enthusiasm."
—Steven Wright

"A word to the wise ain't necessary - it's the stupid ones that need the advice."
—Bill Cosby

Laughter is definitely great medicine for the soul.

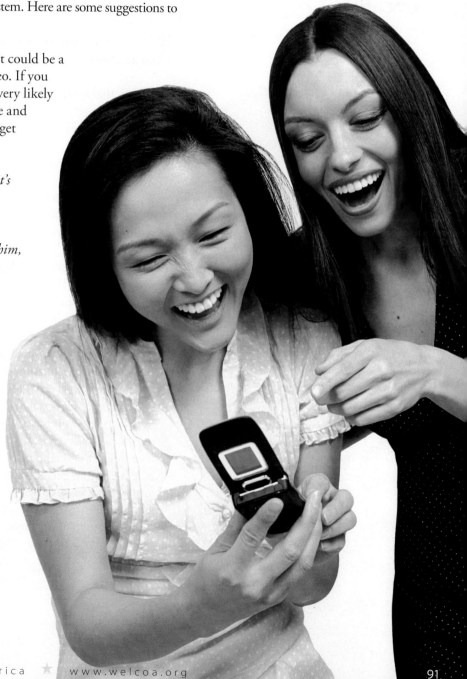

> Emotional well-being is one of the most essential aspects of wellness, yet it is one that gets little attention.

2. Start a tickler notebook. Begin to collect funny jokes, birthday cards, quotes and photos that bring a smile to your face and warm your heart. When you are having a bad day, pull out the tickler notebook and use it to balance your scale of emotions. Here is a joke to begin your tickler notebook: Exercise 5.5 has a few more. Good luck collecting!

The Conversation

God is sitting in heaven when a scientist says to Him, "Lord, we don't need you anymore. Science has finally figured out a way to create life out of nothing. In other words, we can now do what you did in the beginning."

"Is that so? Tell me about it," replies God.

"Well," says the scientist, "we can take dirt and form it into the likeness of You and breathe life into it, thus creating man."

"Well, that's interesting. Show Me."

So the scientist bends down to the earth and starts to mold the soil.

"No, no, no..." interrupts God, "Get your own dirt."

3. Build a humor library of funny cartoon books (e.g. *Calvin and Hobbes, Bizzaro,* etc.). Once you have created your library, make a habit of visiting it on a regular basis.

4. Go see a funny play or musical or go to a comedy club. There are many venues for immediate comic relief right in your locale. Make it a habit to frequent these venues often.

We all know somebody who was a class clown in school. These people love an audience no matter how old they are. Support groups are essential for a merry heart. Sometimes we have to be our own class clown. Exercise 5.6, *Working the Funny Bone,* provides some exercises to get you on your way.

Emotional well-being is one of the most essential aspects of wellness, yet it is one that gets little attention. We ignore our feelings of grief, we wallow in pity, we become easily frustrated, perhaps even depressed at times, we are easily stressed and we forget to appreciate all the good things in life that we take for granted. Make a habit at the end of each day to reflect on all the things in life that are going in your favor. Make a habit to count your blessings.

When all is said and done, it's not about the accumulation of material possessions that provides happiness. It all comes down to the expression of love in all its many colors.

People all over the world have been looking for the secret to success as if it were the Holy Grail (perhaps it is)! This we do know: Success isn't based on job titles or wads of money. Over a hundred years ago, Ralph Waldo Emerson wrote these words and they are as true today as the day he first uttered them:

> *To laugh often and love much; to win the respect of intelligent persons and the affection of children; to earn the approbation of honest citizens and endure the betrayal of false friends; to appreciate beauty; to find the best in others; to give of one's self; to leave the world a bit better, whether by a healthy child, a garden patch or a redeemed social condition; to have played and laughed with enthusiasm and sung with exultation; to know even one life has breathed easier because you have lived—this is to have succeeded.*

66 *This we do know: Success isn't based on job titles or wads of money.* 99

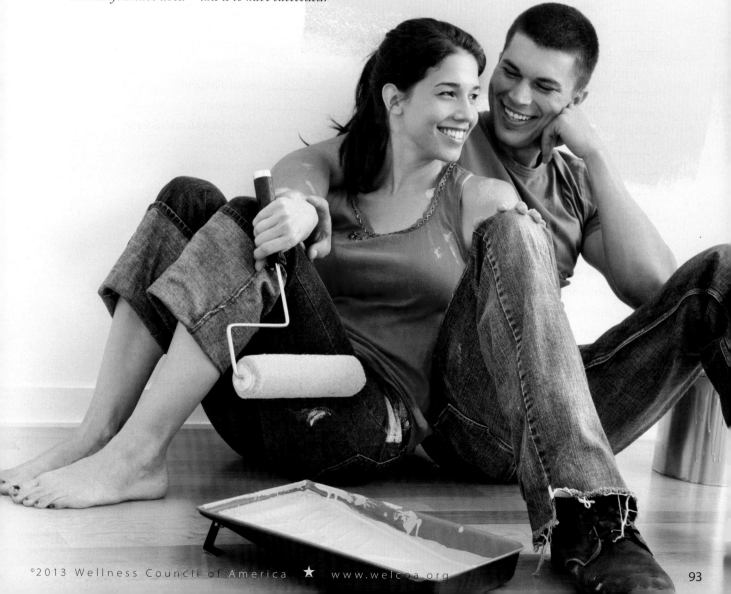

[EXERCISE 5.1]

Anger Recognition Checklist

The following is a quick exercise to help you understand how anger can surface in the course of a normal working day and how you may mismanage it. Please place a checkmark in front of any of the following that apply to you when you get angry or feel frustrated or upset. After completing this section, please refer to the bottom right-hand corner to estimate, on average, the number of anger episodes you experience per day.

When I feel angry, my anger tends to surface in the following ways:

_____ anxious	_____ cry
_____ depressed	_____ threaten others
_____ overeat	_____ buy things
_____ start dieting	_____ frequent lateness
_____ trouble sleeping	_____ never feel angry
_____ excessive sleeping	_____ clenched jaw muscles, TMJD
_____ careless driving	_____ bored
_____ chronic fatigue	_____ nausea, vomiting
_____ abuse alcohol/drugs	_____ skin problems
_____ explode in rage	_____ easily irritable
_____ cold withdrawal	_____ sexual difficulty
_____ tension headaches	_____ sexual apathy
_____ migraine headaches	_____ busy work (clean, straighten)
_____ use sarcasm	_____ sulk, whine
_____ hostile joking	_____ hit, throw things
_____ accident prone	_____ complain, whine
_____ guilty and self-blaming	_____ cut/mutilate myself
_____ smoke or drink	_____ insomnia
_____ high blood pressure	_____ promiscuity
_____ frequent nightmares	_____ help others
_____ tendency to harp or nag	_____ other? _____
_____ intellectualize	_____ other? _____
_____ upset stomach (e.g., gas, cramps, IBS)	
_____ muscle tension (neck, lower back)	*My average number of anger
_____ swear and/or name call	episodes per day is _____

> " He who angers you, conquers you. "
>
> —Elizabeth Kenny

[EXERCISE 5.2]

Mismanaged Anger Style Indicator

PART I: Check the statements that are true for you the majority of the time.

_____ 1. Even though I may wish to complain, I usually don't.

_____ 2. When upset, I have a habit of slamming, punching, or breaking things.

_____ 3. When I feel guilty, I have been known to contemplate self-destructive behaviors.

_____ 4. I can be real nice to people, but then back-stab them when they're not around.

_____ 5. I have a habit of grinding my teeth at night.

_____ 6. When I am really irritated or frustrated by others, I tend to intimidate them.

_____ 7. When I am frustrated, I feel like going shopping and spending money.

_____ 8. I can manipulate people without them even knowing it.

_____ 9. It's fair to say that I rarely, if ever, get angry or mad.

_____ 10. I have been known to talk back to people of authority.

_____ 11. Sleeping in is a good way to forget about my problems and frustrations.

_____ 12. Watching TV or playing video games offers a good escape from my frustrations.

_____ 13. If I complain, I feel people won't like me as much, so I usually don't.

_____ 14. When driving at times, I feel like I want to hit people with my car.

_____ 15. When I get mad or frustrated, I have been known to eat to calm my nerves.

_____ 16. I plan a script or rehearse what I am going to say to win a conflict.

_____ 17. Its hard/uncomfortable for me to say the words "I am angry."

_____ 18. I usually try to get the final say in situations with others.

_____ 19. I have been known to use alcohol and/or drugs to deal with my angry feelings.

_____ 20. By and large, I tend to agree with the statement, "Don't get mad, get even."

_____ 21. I tend to keep my feelings to myself.

_____ 22. When I get angry, I have been known to swear a lot.

_____ 23. I usually feel guilty about feeling angry, frustrated, or annoyed.

_____ 24. It's OK to use sarcasm to make a point.

_____ 25. I am the kind of person who calms the waters when tempers flare at home or work.

_____ 26. It's easy to say the words "I am angry" or "I am pissed" and really mean it.

_____ 27. On more than one occasion, I have imagined taking my own life.

_____ 28. I think of various ways to put people down.

_____ 29. Typically, I place the needs of others before myself.

_____ 30. I suffer from migraine headaches or TMJD or rheumatoid arthritis or lupus.

PART II: SCORE SHEET- Write down the numbers of the statement that you checked off in Part I:

_____

We all tend to engage in all of these behaviors at some time; however, some behaviors are very common to us whereas others are more occasional, suggesting that when certain predominant behaviors are grouped together they reveal a specific style of mismanaged anger. Mismanaged anger leads to a host of serious problems for both you and others. By learning to recognize the series of behaviors that fall into one or perhaps two categories, you can more easily identify behavior patterns and then implement strategies to address and modify those patterns. Labels are good to identify behaviors, but they are not meant to serve as mismanaged "scarlet letters."

> If you have four or more answers from: 1, 5, 9, 13, 17, 21, 25, 29, or 30, your mismanaged anger style strongly suggests you might be a Somatizer (Silent-But- Deadly Stone).

> If you have four or more answers from: 2, 6, 10, 14, 18, 22, or 26, your mismanaged anger style strongly suggests you might be an Exploder (Volcanic Stone).

> If you have four or more answers from: 3, 7, 11, 12, 15, 19, 23, or 27, your mismanaged anger style strongly suggests you might be a Self-Punisher (Razor Stone).

> If you have four or more answers from: 4, 8, 16, 20, 24, or 28 your mismanaged anger style strongly suggests you might be an Underhander (Revenge Stone).

[FIGURE 5.1]

Mismanaged Anger Cycle (Picking Up Hot Stones)

Metaphorically speaking, anger is said to be like a hot stone. The mismanaged anger cycle begins with the interpretation of some event [#1] (internal or external) and progresses clockwise [#2]—[#5] in an unbroken circle of anger (frustration to rage) where anger feelings begin and are perpetuated because they are not resolved. Anger as a hot stone…burns!

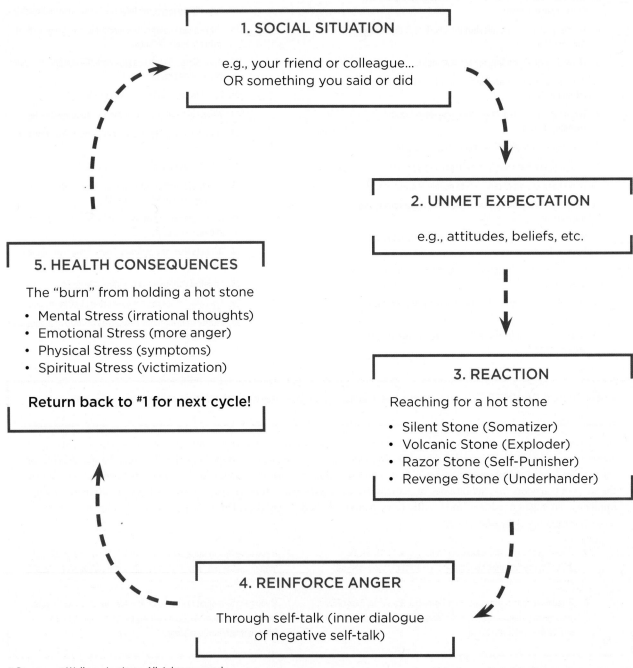

1. SOCIAL SITUATION

e.g., your friend or colleague…
OR something you said or did

2. UNMET EXPECTATION

e.g., attitudes, beliefs, etc.

5. HEALTH CONSEQUENCES

The "burn" from holding a hot stone

- Mental Stress (irrational thoughts)
- Emotional Stress (more anger)
- Physical Stress (symptoms)
- Spiritual Stress (victimization)

Return back to #1 for next cycle!

3. REACTION

Reaching for a hot stone

- Silent Stone (Somatizer)
- Volcanic Stone (Exploder)
- Razor Stone (Self-Punisher)
- Revenge Stone (Underhander)

4. REINFORCE ANGER

Through self-talk (inner dialogue
of negative self-talk)

[FIGURE 5.2]

Strategies For Well-Managed Anger (Dropping Hot Stones)

In a well-managed anger style, the cycle of anger is broken because the situation and the feelings generated from it are worked through and resolved starting with #1 and ending with #5.

1. CONFLICT SITUATION

Anger feelings begin (e.g., impatience, envy, guilt, rage)

2. IDENTIFY UNMET EXPECTATIONS & RECOGNIZE & VALIDATE YOUR FEELINGS

Remember, it's OK (normal) to "feel" angry

3. EVALUATE THE SITUATION:

Why are my thoughts irrational?

Do I have all the information I need to understand the situation?

What expectations weren't met?

4. BE PROACTIVE NOT REACTIVE! EXHIBIT CONTROL!

1. Do not pick up a hot stone.

2. Drop the hot stone you may have already picked up in defense.

3. Use auditory, visual and kinetic strategies to re-script the irrational thoughts and negative self-talk.

5. PROBLEM RESOLUTION

Positively resolve the conflict (use one or more coping strategies)

[EXERCISE 5.3]

Creative Anger Management Skills Action Plan

Dealing with anger effectively means working to resolve the issues and expectations that surfaced from the anger episode. There are many ways to creatively resolve anger so that you reclaim your emotional sovereignty. The following is a synthesis of suggestions from a variety of sources. Read through each suggestion and below it write a description of what steps you can implement to creatively manage your anger and keep each episode of anger within a healthy time period.

1. **Know your anger style -** What is your most predominant mismanaged anger style?

_____

2. **Learn to self-monitor your anger -** Reflect on the past day's events (including listening to the news) and estimate the number of times you felt anger:

_____

3. **Learn to de-escalate your anger -** List three ways to let off steam (e.g., leave the room, take a big sigh, count to ten):

    1. _____
    2. _____
    3. _____

4. **Learn to out-think your anger -** Many times anger results from insufficient information. Identify an anger situation and re-process the information to neutralize your anger feelings:

_____

5. **Get comfortable with all your feelings -** Some people have a hard time saying the phrase, "I am angry," or "I feel angry." Are you one of them? Please explain.

_____

6. **Plan in advance -** Although avoidance is not advocated, making plans to work around a problem is known as the path of least resistance. Identify a current frustration and then list three things you can do as an action plan to rise above the occasion!

    1. _____
    2. _____
    3. _____

7. **Develop a strong support system -** List three people whom you can turn to vent your frustrations as well as who can provide an objective voice about your stressful situation.

    1. _____
    2. _____
    3. _____

8. **Develop realistic expectations for yourself and others -** Pick one anger situation you have had today (or yesterday), identify the expectation that wasn't met, and then refine the expectation.

    Unmet expectation: _____

    Refined expectation: _____

9. **Turn complaints into requests -** As the expression goes, you get more flies with honey than vinegar. Script a phrase that you can use to incorporate the magic of request.

_____

10. **Make past anger pass -** Letting go of anger begins with forgiveness. List three people whom you feel have violated you in some way, and who still need your forgiveness to bring closure to the situation.

    1. _____
    2. _____
    3. _____

[EXERCISE 5.4]

1,000 Things Went Right Today!®

In a stress-filled world, it becomes easy to start focusing on the negative things in life. Pretty soon you begin to attract more negative things in your life. Breaking free from this thought process isn't easy, but it's not impossible. There is an expression coined by Ilan Shamir which states, "A thousand things went right today."® The concept behind this expression suggests that by beginning to look for the positive things in life, you will start attracting positive things, and let's face it, we can all use more positivity in our lives. Rather than taxing your mind to come up with 1,000 things or even 100, try starting with 10 things that went right today, and then see if you can begin to include this frame of mind at the midpoint of each day to keep on course. Remember, in a world of negativity, it takes work to be happy!

1. _____

2. _____

3. _____

4. _____

5. _____

6. _____

7. _____

8. _____

9. _____

10. _____

After having written down these things, is there any lesson that comes to mind that you can learn from this experience?

_____

_____

_____

_____

_____

_____

[EXERCISE 5.5]

Making A Tickler Notebook

Consider this! The average child laughs or giggles about 300 times a day. The typical adult laughs about 15 times a day. Research reveals that the average hospital patient never laughs at all. This assignment invites you to make a tickler notebook (3-ring notebooks work best) comprised of favorite jokes, photographs, birthday cards, love letters, Dear Abby columns, poems or anything else that brings a smile to your face. Keep the tickler notebook on hand so if you are having a bad day, you can pull it out to help you regain some emotional balance. And, if you ever find yourself in the hospital for whatever reason, be sure to bring it along so that you can at least get your quota of 15 laughs a day. The following are two jokes to help you form a critical mass of funny things to include in your notebook.

The New Boss:

A company, feeling it is time for a shakeup, hires a new CEO. This new boss is determined to rid the company of all slackers. On a tour of the facilities, the CEO notices a guy leaning on a wall. The room is full of workers and he wants to let them know he means business! The CEO walks up to the guy and asks, "And how much money do you make a week?" Undaunted, the young fellow looks at him and replies, "I make about $200 a week. Why?"

The CEO hands the guy $1,000 in cash and screams, "Here's a month's pay with benefits, now GET OUT and don't come back!"

Surprisingly, the guy takes the cash with a smile, says "Yes sir! Thank you, sir!" and leaves.

Feeling pretty good about his first firing, the CEO looks around the room and asks, "Does anyone want to tell me what that slacker did around here?"

With a sheepish grin, one of the other workers mutters, "Pizza delivery guy from Domino's."

Welcome To The Bell Curve Of Life:

At age 4, success is…   not peeing in your pants.
At age 12, success is…   having friends.
At age 16, success is…   having a driver's license.
At age 20, success is…   having sex.
At age 30, success is…   having money.
At age 50, success is…   having money.
At age 60, success is…   having sex.
At age 70, success is…   having a driver's license.
At age 75, success is…   having friends.
At age 80, success is…   not peeing in your pants!

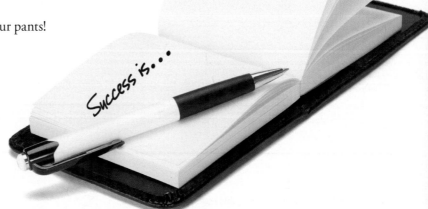

[EXERCISE 5.6]

Working The Funny Bone

1. It's time to create a new answering machine message. Most likely your answering machine message is the same as everyone else's. Here is an example of a winning voice mail message. See if you can come up with something equally funny:

    Hi, you've reached the home of Bob and Jill. We can't come to the phone right now because we are doing something we really enjoy. Jill likes doing it up and down. I like doing it sideways. Just as soon as we get done brushing our teeth, we'll call you right back.

    Your new voice mail message:

    _____
    _____
    _____

2. Humor means "fluid" or "moisture" so let the juice flow! Complete the following sentence by filling in the blank. Combine your talents of creativity and exaggeration to come up with something funny.

    You know you're having a bad day when:

    _____
    _____
    _____

3. You (or a good friend) are new in town and are looking for a new romantic relationship. The problem is shyness, so the solution is a personal ad. Remember that a sense of humor is one of the first things people look for in a "mate." Write your personal ad:

    _____
    _____
    _____

4. You are a vaudevillian songwriter who has been asked to write some new lyrics for the chorus of one of these commonly known songs. Parody a topic (e.g., health care problems, political characters, environmental problems, any news headline).

    a. Home on the Range   d. My Favorite Things
    b. Our House   e. A rap song
    c. Cabaret   f. Your choice

5. Make a list of your top five movie comedies (with the intention of seeing them again soon):

    1. _____
    2. _____
    3. _____
    4. _____
    5. _____

[CHAPTER 6]

Spiritual Well-Being

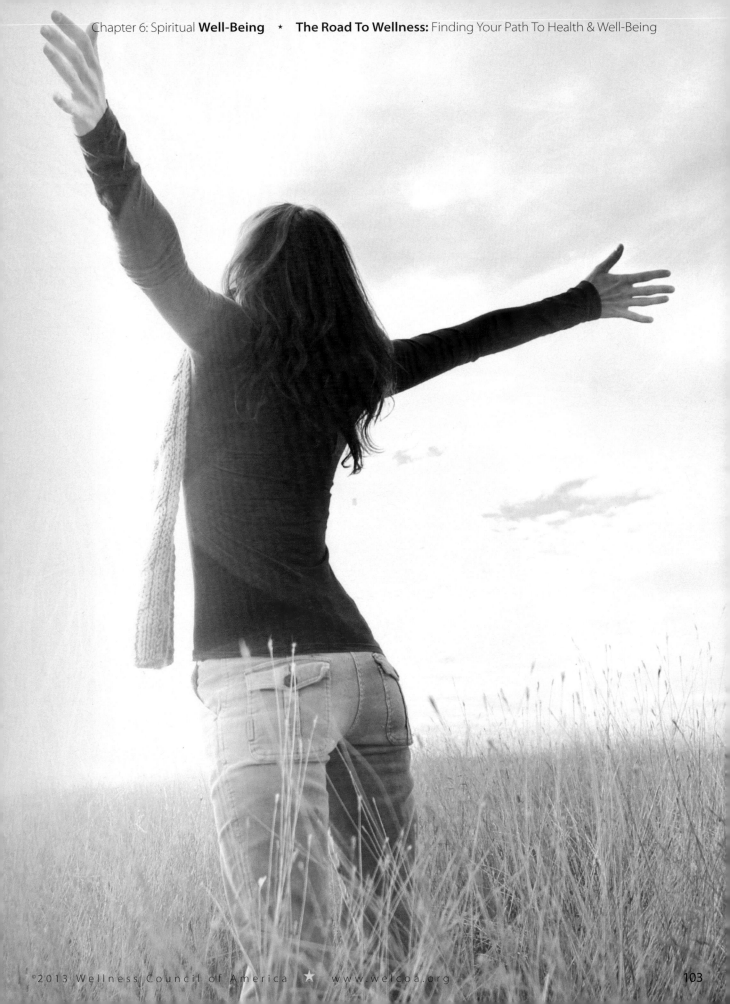

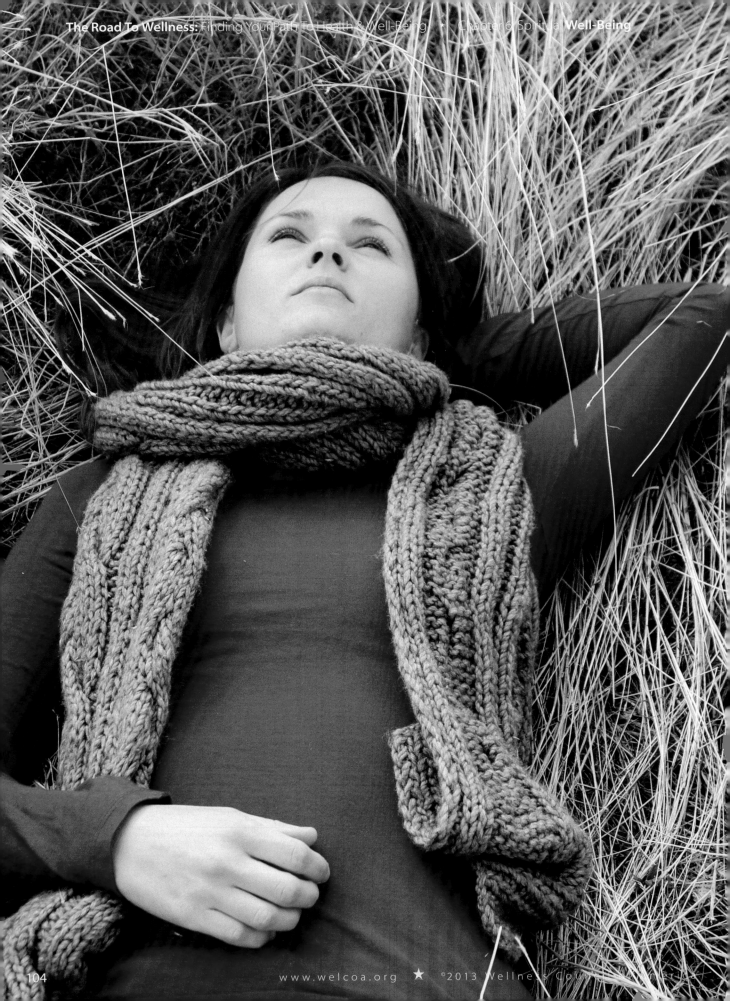

[CHAPTER 6]

Spiritual Well-Being

The triumph of the human spirit is a story that never grows old. Nelson Mandela. Mahatma Gandhi. Jews who survived the atrocities of Nazi concentration camps. Rosa Parks. Boston area residents and marathon runners. A multitude of cancer patients who face death gracefully. Aaron Ralston. Returning war soldiers, Antarctic explorer Ernest Shackleton and countless other heroes whose names may be less recognizable, but whose stories are equally impressive. It is these remarkable stories that serve as both map and compass for our own life journey because life indeed is challenging, if not incredibly difficult at times. When we hear of someone who has overcome adversity, someone who has beaten the unlikely odds and come home the victor, a part of us celebrates too. The triumph of the human spirit is the epitome of strong spiritual well-being; the health of the human spirit. Although much neglected and often ignored, spiritual well-being is the cornerstone of personal wellness.

There are two ways to face adversity. The first way is to declare yourself a victim and give up. Sadly, many people do this all too often. Not only does this story quickly become boring, but it ultimately serves no greater purpose. Nazi concentration camp survivor Gerta Weisman Klein has this to say about this approach, "Giving up is the final solution to a temporary

> *Although much neglected and often ignored, spiritual well-being is the cornerstone of personal wellness.*

problem." The second way, the preferred option, is to forge ahead, no matter the odds and come through as the victor. Not only are these people heroes; they prove to be excellent role models and teachers. Quite often when these people are asked to share their personal stories, they often say this: "At the time I was going through this ordeal, I thought it was the worst thing that could ever happen to me. Now, I can honestly say, it was the best thing that ever happened to me." These words bring to mind the famous quote uttered by Winston Churchill during World War II: "If you are going through hell... keep going!"

The Cornerstone And Foundation Of Human Spirituality

If you were to talk to the shamans, sages, mystics and healers of all times, all cultures and all languages and ask them what is the core essence of human spirituality, they would tell you this: human spirituality is the maturation of higher consciousness as expressed through three facets: relationships, values and a meaningful purpose in life. Moreover, these same wisdom keepers would tell you that while human spirituality and religion share common ground, they are not the same thing. You can be spiritual but not religious, just as you can be religious but not spiritual. Spirituality is experiential and very personal. Your spiritual experiences, whatever they may happen to be, will undoubtedly be quite different than anyone else's. Yet, at the same time, each of these experiences reminds us that we are part of something much, much bigger (whatever you consider this to be). The world does not revolve around us. In the words of poet Maya Angelou, "I believe that spirit is one and everywhere present. That it never leaves me. I may withdraw from it, but I can realize its presence the instant I return to my senses. I cannot separate what I conceive as spirit from my concept of God." Exercise 6.1 offers you the opportunity to take a personal look at the three pillars of human spirituality; relationships, values and a meaningful purpose in life.

The Hero's Journey

Several decades ago, a young man from New York named Joseph Campbell took a deep interest in the fables and stories of American Indians. This fascination soon led him to explore a treasure-trove of ancient myths and legends from cultures all around the world—from Egypt and India to the Tlingit tribe of Sitka, Alaska. In hearing all these stories he had a realization. All good stories have more than just a beginning, middle and end. Mythical stories have a template that describes the plight of the human journey; a journey he called the Hero's Journey.

Campbell found that every great story has three parts; 1) the departure; going from the known into the unknown, 2) the initiation; accomplishing a specific and difficult task or assignment, and, 3) the return home where the hero not only celebrates the victory, but shares what was learned on the journey so that all may benefit from this wisdom. Home is a metaphor for homeostasis or inner peace; the resolution of the problem. The Hero's Journey is the spiritual journey. It is a journey that we all participate in because the Hero's Journey is the journey of life.

> ...human spirituality is the maturation of higher consciousness as expressed through three facets: relationships, values and a meaningful purpose in life.

Campbell studied the stories of ancient Greek, Roman, Norwegian and Asian mythology, yet even contemporary stories follow the same template: Dorothy had quite the departure out of Kansas. Her initiation was to get the broomstick from the Wicked Witch of the West, and all it took to get home was the click of those ruby red slippers. Frodo didn't want to leave the Shire, but off he went to Mount Doom to get rid of the ring. He made it back home safely too (minus a finger). Luke Skywalker, Ariel the mermaid, Jason and the Argonauts, Spider-Man, even James Bond and Lucy Ricardo (*I Love Lucy*) are all classic heroic characters with one message. You too can make it back home safely. We need to hear these messages because so often in the struggle of daily life we become distracted or worse, get lost and cannot find our way home easily.

How long is the Hero's Journey? Perhaps it cannot be measured! Yet there are those who certainly try. But this we know: the spiritual path cannot be measured in miles. It also cannot be measured in possessions, but boy do we try. It's quite possible that it can be measured in personal experiences, though some might disagree. There are a select few who say that the spiritual path is between 12 to 14 inches; the distance from your head to your heart.

How is your Journey going? Exercise 6.2 invites you to take a closer look at the plot of your own life through the lens of The Hero's Journey.

Muscles Of The Soul

When the police knocked on her front door, Rose immediately knew something was wrong. In fact, you might say she was expecting them. Call it a mother's intuition. The lead officer invited himself in and asked Rose to have a seat, whereupon he informed her that her 22 year old son, Ben, had been killed in a car accident less than an hour previous; killed by a drunk driver. One of the hardest things in the world to experience is the loss of a child. Rose was devastated, completing devastated. "When your life crumbles, you have two choices: let the wind blow you around aimlessly or raise your sails and use these winds of change to your advantage," she said. "I was angry at this guy who killed my son. But I knew the anger would consume me if I let it. I had to let it go. The only answer was forgiveness. Several months later, on the day of the defendant's court appearance, I read a statement to the judge asking for leniency. It was the hardest thing I have ever had to do, but I knew in my heart I had to do it. I know that my life is better for it," she explained.

> *...the spiritual path cannot be measured in miles.*

> *The spiritual path is well marked with peaks and valleys, winding curves and long stretches of vast expanse.*

Human beings have a most remarkable tool kit to deal with adversity. Psychologists call these tools "inner resources." Some people call them coping skills. Joseph Campbell used the term "the assistance of spiritual aids." They also go by the expression "muscles of the soul." When people who have faced such adversity are asked how they overcame it, they often describe these inner resources as paramount to their success. These muscles are not gifts for a chosen few; they are birthrights for everyone. Like our physical muscles (e.g., biceps, deltoids, quadriceps, etc.) these spiritual muscles will never simply disappear, but they will atrophy with disuse. Here is a short list: Patience, courage, humor, forgiveness, optimism, persistence, faith, tolerance, honesty, creativity, intuition, humbleness, curiosity, integrity, resiliency and compassion. These inner resources are not Christian, Jewish, Islamic, Taoist, or Shinto resources. They are human resources. It is these muscles of the soul that help the hero dismantle, circumnavigate or transcend the roadblocks (more commonly called stressors) and move on with our lives gracefully and return home. These muscles need to be exercised regularly. One final note: Campbell reminds us that there is not one but many journeys in the life of a hero. How strong are your spiritual muscles? Exercise 6.3 offers some insight in ways you can work to improve your spiritual potential by flexing these muscles of the soul.

Distractions And Roadblocks On The Path

In a great many languages around the world, the word spirit means breath or wind. The word "spirit" symbolizes a movement of energy (e.g., inhalation followed by exhalation). Even the word "inspired" has a spiritual connotation to it and for good reason. It is inspiration that helps us get through the tough times, as well as a long day at the office. Along the spiritual path, the hero will surely encounter roadblocks and obstructions (part of the initiation process). And while our first inclination is to turn our back and head in another direction, avoidance is never a good coping strategy. As we mature into adulthood, we begin to realize that these roadblocks are actually part of the spiritual path, and they are meant to be resolved, not avoided.

The spiritual path is well marked with peaks and valleys, winding curves and long stretches of vast expanse. It is also filled with lots of distractions; things that pull us off the path and keep us off for quite a while. As the expression goes, it's okay to stop and smell the roses (this is even encouraged) but no one said stop and pull off the road and park for 20 years. Classic fables and stories serve as reminders, if not dire warnings of these distractions. Rip van Winkle comes to mind quite easily. So does the story of Pinocchio. Distractions begin as attractions. A beer is an attraction. Alcoholism is a distraction. It is safe to say that our biggest health issues today include distractions on the spiritual path. For more insight on roadblocks and distractions, please consider completing exercises 6.4 and 6.5.

Seasons Of The Soul

If you were to talk to these same wisdom keepers and ask them about the human journey, you would hear them speak of a concept called the Seasons of the Soul; a process of personal growth and expanded consciousness. Like the earth's seasons, we too have four seasons that we travel through on our human journey, and they nicely parallel the earth's seasons. Here is a closer look:

The Centering Process (Autumn): A soul-searching process, a time to go within and focus on the self. It is a time of self-reflection where one quiets the mind to calm the soul. It is a time to be still. The word center means to "enter the heart." It is similar to the autumn season as with less light one goes inside earlier. In our western-based culture, rich in media smart phones and tablets, we are not encouraged for much self-reflection. The centering process reminds us to take time to go inside.

The Emptying Process (Winter): This is a time to release, let go, and detach from thoughts, attitudes, beliefs and perceptions, which at one time may have served us, but now they no longer do. In fact, they only seem to hold us back. This season goes by many names including the "dark night of the soul" and the "winter of discontent." The dark night, however, is only supposed to be a night, not an eternity. Moreover, this is the one season people tend to avoid. As a consequence, they often get stuck, also known as spiritual constipation. The emptying process is not a pit of despair, it is the womb of creation, but we must take that first step into the void to let go.

The Grounding Process (Spring): A time to seek and process the answers to life's problems and challenges. Followed by the emptying process where things are cleared out, remember that nature abhors a vacuum. Not all insights come immediately. Patience is necessary. Sometimes we must wait for an insight; however, the grounding process is augmented by cultivating the silence of the mind. By making space in the Emptying Process, new insights or wisdom will make itself known to you. When the pupil is ready, the teacher will come. The grounding process is time to access our intuition and perhaps even attain a feeling of enlightenment in preparation for the next stage (season) of our life journey. This insight, this nugget of wisdom is the vision of the vision quest. But remember, greed is not a spiritual value. This wisdom must be shared.

The Connecting Process (Summer): A season when we come back "home" to our community and share what we have learned on the leg of our most recent experience and the wisdom gained from the grounding process. The Connecting Process is based on the premise of love—nurturing our connections with friends, family and acquaintances (even strangers). As such, the Connecting Process is a time of celebration. Careful though, many people tend to get stuck here too!

> what makes life challenging, if not difficult at times, is that we are experiencing different seasons with different life aspects (problems).

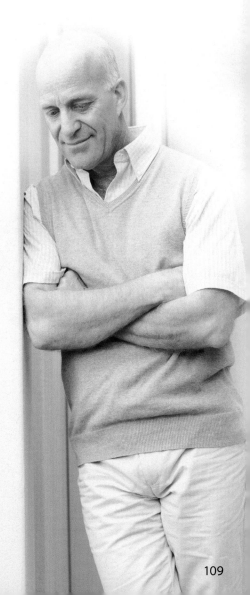

> Sometimes we need to hear the same message different ways before we get it."

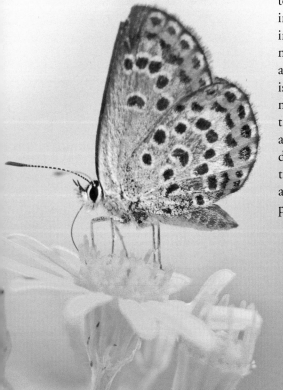

What makes life challenging, if not difficult at times, is that we are experiencing different seasons with different life aspects (problems). For instance, we may be in the emptying process in one aspect of our lives (e.g., career) while smack in the middle of the connecting process for another (e.g., daughter's wedding). Matters become more complex when a loved one (e.g., spouse, friend) experiencing the same situation (e.g., the death of a child) is in one season, while we are in another.

By now you may have noticed that the seasons of the soul are very similar to the stages of the Hero's Journey. There is a good reason. Sometimes we need to hear the same message different ways before we get it. Moreover, the language of spiritual well-being is a difficult one, which is why it is rich in metaphors. Exercise 6.5 offers you another look at your life through the template of these seasons.

Health Of The Human Spirit

How does one cultivate the health of the human spirit? There are many ways. Breathing in the beauty of a crimson sunset. Expressing a heartfelt apology. Offering gratitude for the beauty of a monarch butterfly. Performing a random act of kindness. Acknowledging the reassuring voice of a good friend. These are gifts that nurture the soul. We yearn for and cherish these special moments to give balance to that which so often and so easily becomes off-balance through the hectic demands and increasing pressures of our jobs, families and uncalculated events in everyday life. These gifts; a type of divine energy, so to speak, filter through our senses to invigorate the human spirit; the essence of life that seeks to resonate in every cell in our body. And in cyclical fashion, it is the vibrancy of our inner resources (e.g., honesty, forgiveness, patience and love), which like a magnet, continually draws our attention toward these special moments. This awareness that recognizes the unique alchemy of humanity and divinity is that which allows us to best cope with life's problems. Moreover, this mystical alchemy which sustains the health of the human spirit is none other than the most sound strategy for optimal wellness because it acknowledges and honors, rather than ignores the critical importance of the spiritual dimension. Let us not forget that one of the most important ways to nurture the health of the human spirit is to resolve issues of anger and fear. If you are still looking for ways to cultivate a stronger sense of spiritual well-being, please consider completing exercise 6.7, *Health of the Human Spirit*.

[EXERCISE 6.1]

The Three Pillars Of Human Spirituality

The shamans, healers, sages, and wisdom keepers of all times, all continents, and all peoples, in their ageless wisdom say that human spirituality is composed of three aspects: relationships, values and purpose in life. These three components are so tightly integrated that it may be hard to separate them from each other. But if this were possible, take a moment to reflect on these aspects of human spirituality to determine the status of your spiritual well-being.

I. Relationships - All life is a relationship! In simple terms, there are two categories of relationships: internal (your domestic policy); how you deal with yourself, how you nurture the relationship with yourself and your higher-self, and external relationships (your foreign policy); how you relate, support and interact with those people in your environment. How would you evaluate your internal relationship and what steps could you take to cultivate it? Moving from the aspect of "domestic policy" to "foreign policy" how would you evaluate your external relationships?

_____

_____

_____

_____

II. Your Personal Value System - We each have a value system composed of core and supporting values. Core values (about 4 to 6) are those which form the foundation of our personal belief system. Supporting values support the core values. Intangible core values (e.g., love, honesty, freedom) and supporting values (e.g., education, creativity and integrity) are often symbolized in material possessions. Quite regularly, our personal value system tends to go through a reorganization process, particularly when there are conflicts in our values. What are your core and supporting values? Please list them below.

Core Values
1. _____
2. _____
3. _____
4. _____
5. _____

Supporting Values
1. _____
2. _____
3. _____
4. _____
5. _____

III. A Meaningful Purpose In Life - A meaningful purpose in life is that which gives our life meaning. Some might call it a life mission. Although it is true that we may have an overall life mission, it is also true that our lives are a collection of meaningful purposes. Suffering waits in those times in between each purpose. What would you say is your life mission and what purpose are you now supporting to accomplish this mission?

_____

_____

_____

_____

_____

Every crisis over the age of 30 is a spiritual crisis. Spiritual crises require spiritual cures.

—Carl Gustav Jung

[EXERCISE 6.2]

The Hero's Journey
Exploring The Wisdom Of Joseph Campbell

An ancient proverb states, "It takes a brave soul to walk the planet earth." In the eyes of the divine, we are all heroes. The role of a hero is not an easy one. To depart from home can promote feelings of insecurity and even abandonment. Initiations, and there are many in one lifetime, are demanding and arduous; the phrase "baptism by fire" comes to mind. Yet through it all we are assured a warm reception upon our return, no matter the outcome of our journey.

The Hero's Journey is a mythical quest. Myths are clues to the spiritual potential of human life. They offer meaning and significance as well as values. A myth is a source of truth, which often becomes exaggerated, but still holds its own essence. According to Campbell (who filmed a PBS special called *The Power of Myth*), a myth does four things to assist us on this remarkable journey:

1. A myth brings us into communion with the transcendent realms and eternal forms.

2. A myth provides a revelation to waking consciousness of the power of its sustaining source.

3. A myth tells us that no matter the culture, the rituals of living and dying have spiritual and moral roots.

4. A myth fosters the centering and unfolding of the individual in integrity with the ultimate creative mystery that is both beyond and within oneself and all things.

Campbell was of the opinion that the greatest danger of the Hero's Journey is to fail to use the power of myth as a guide on the spiritual path. He was keenly aware that the contemporary American culture has abandoned its association with myths, a clear and present danger to any society.

The Spiritual Quest: Your Mythical Journey
The plot of every myth includes a beginning, a middle and an end. In this case, the beginning is a departure from the known and familiar, the middle is a set of trials (called initiations) and the end is the return back home. In truth, we engage in this process of the Hero's Journey many times during the course of our lives.

1. **The Departure:** Are you in the process of moving out of the familiar into the unknown? What are you departing from? For some people, there is a refusal of the call. This is often based on some fear of the unknown. Are you ignoring a call to move on?

_____
_____
_____
_____

2. **The Initiation:** The initiation is the threshold of adventure. Mythically speaking, the initiation is to slay a dragon or monster. In real life, initiations come in many forms, from rites of passage to issues, problems and stressors. What is the single major life issue, concern, or problem that you are facing at the present moment?

_____
_____
_____
_____

3. The Return Home: The return is symbolized by coming home; home to the old life but with a fresh perspective. The return home bears a responsibility of sharing what you have learned on the journey. What have you learned from your most recent journey?

_____

_____

_____

_____

4. A Working Myth: What myth (source of truth) do you hold as a compass on your spiritual quest? Where did you learn this myth and how has it helped you in your life?

_____

_____

_____

_____

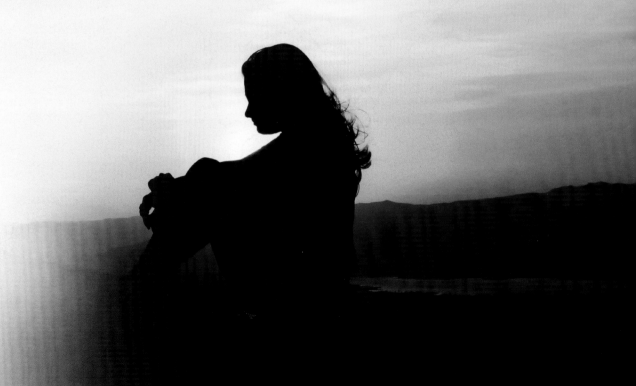

[EXERCISE 6.3]

Muscles Of The Soul
Exploring The Wisdom Of Joseph Campbell

Just as a circle is a universal symbol of wholeness, so too is the butterfly a symbol of wholeness. Given the fact that butterflies, unlike the lowly caterpillar, have wings to fly, butterflies also are considered a symbol of transformation. They can rise above what was once considered a limiting existence. There is a story of a boy who, upon seeing a young butterfly trying to emerge from its chrysalis, tried to help by pulling apart the paper cocoon that housed the metamorphosis. The boy's mother who saw what he was about to do quickly stopped him by explaining that the butterfly strengthens its young wings by pushing through the walls of the cocoon. In doing so, its wings become strong enough to fly.

If you were to talk with anyone who has emerged gracefully from a difficult situation, they would most likely tell you that the muscles they used to break through their barrier(s) included patience, humor, forgiveness, optimism, humbleness, creativity, persistence, courage, willpower and love. Some people call these inner resources. I call these "muscles of the soul." These are the muscles we use to dismantle, circumnavigate, and transcend the roadblocks and obstacles in life. Like physical muscles, these muscles will never disappear; however, they will atrophy with disuse. We are given ample opportunity to exercise these muscles, yet not everyone does.

Using the butterfly illustration, write in the wings those attributes, inner resources and muscles of the soul that you feel help you get through the tough times—with grace and dignity, rather than feeling victimized. If there are traits you wish to include to augment the health of your human spirit, yet you feel aren't quite there, write those outside the wings and then draw an arrow into the wings, giving your soul a message that you wish to include (strengthen) these as well. Finally, if you have a box of crayons or pastels, color in your butterfly. Then hang it up on the fridge or bathroom mirror—some place where you can see it regularly to remind yourself of your spiritual health and your innate ability to transcend life's problems, both big and small.

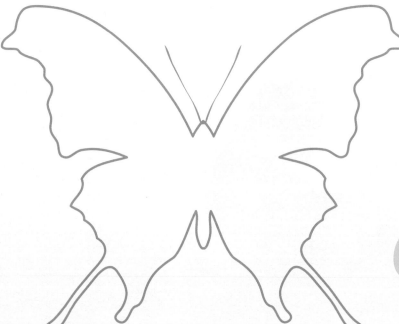

Giving up is the final solution to a temporary problem.

—Gerta Weisman Klein,
Nazi concentration camp survivor

[EXERCISE 6.4]

Roadblocks On The Human Path

If our experience on the human path is indeed the evolution of our soul growth process, then roadblocks can metaphorically be used to describe a temporary halt to this evolutionary process. Roadblocks on the human path are not necessarily aspects in our lives that separate us from our divine source or mission—even though they may seem like this at times. Rather, roadblocks are part of the human path. And while they may initially seem to stifle or inhibit our spiritual growth, this only occurs if we give up or give in to them and do nothing. In the words of a Nazi concentration camp Holocaust survivor, "Giving up is a final solution to a temporary problem."

Roadblocks take many forms, including unresolved anger or fear, greed, apathy, laziness, excessive judgment, and denial, just to name a few. More often than not, these obstacles manifest symbolically as problems, issues, and concerns (and sometimes people). Although the first thing we may want to do when coming upon a roadblock is retreat and do an about-face, avoidance only serves to postpone the inevitable. Miles down the road we will encounter the same obstacles. Roadblocks must be dealt with.

First make a list of what you consider to be some of the major (tangible) obstacles on your human journey (e.g., the boss from hell, the ex-spouse from hell, etc.) Take a moment to identify each with a sentence or two.

1. _____
_____
2. _____
_____
3. _____
_____
4. _____
_____
5. _____
_____

Next, begin to ask yourself to identify what emotions are associated with each roadblock just listed. What emotions do they elicit, and why do you suppose these emotions surface for you as these obstacles come into view?

1. _____
_____
2. _____
_____
3. _____
_____
4. _____
_____
5. _____
_____

[EXERCISE 6.5]

Distractions On The Human Path

Distractions can best be described as those things that pull us off the spiritual path—indefinitely. Distractions begin as attractions, but the allure can often cast a spell of slumber on the soul growth process. Although a respite on the human journey is desirable and even necessary at times, a prolonged distraction will ultimately weaken our spiritual resolve. The human spirit, like energy, must flow and never stagnate.

The lessons of distractions are quite common in fairy tales. Whether it is the story of Pinocchio or Hansel and Gretel, the warnings regarding distractions are as plentiful as the distractions themselves. The lessons of distractions are common in the great spiritual teachings as well. Here they are called temptations. Not always, but often, attractions that become distractions have an addictive quality to them as well.

What happens when we become distracted? Metaphorically speaking, we fall asleep on the human path. Like Dorothy and her friends on the way to Oz who stepped off the yellow brick road to smell the poppies and fell fast asleep, we too lose our direction, our mission, and our energy stagnates. The end result is never promising.

Unlike roadblocks, distractions are not so much meant to be circumvented, dismantled or even transcended. Rather, they are meant to be appreciated—perhaps from afar, perhaps enjoyed briefly and then left behind. Fairy tales aside, what are contemporary distractions? Common day examples of every day distractions might include social contacts, alcohol, television, cell phones, and the Internet.

Take a moment to reflect on what might be some distractions in your life. Make a list and describe each one in a sentence or two. Upon recognition of these, what steps can you take to "wake up" and get back on the path?

1. _____
_____

2. _____
_____

3. _____
_____

4. _____
_____

5. _____
_____

[EXERCISE 6.6]

Your Seasons Of The Soul

Centering, emptying, grounding and connecting constitute the four seasons of the soul. Now is the time to take stock of your life. Are you in the midst of one particular season at the present time? Like the planet earth, we can have many seasons occurring at the same time. There is a normal procession of these seasons, however, it is easy to get stuck in one particular season of the soul. The emptying process is one season most people try to avoid only to remain stuck there the longest. Based on the concepts explained earlier in this chapter, take a moment to identify where you feel you are at this time in your life. Please identify what you normally do in each season to get the most out of it. Is there a season you choose to skip? If so, why? Do you take periodic time to do some quality soul searching? Of these four seasons, is there one that seems to hold the most importance for you? If so, why? How would you describe your connecting process?

The Centering Process (Autumn)

_____
_____
_____
_____
_____

The Emptying Process (Winter)

_____
_____
_____
_____
_____

The Grounding Process (Spring)

_____
_____
_____
_____
_____

The Connecting Process (Summer)

_____
_____
_____
_____
_____

[EXERCISE 6.7]

Health Of The Human Spirit

Imagine, if you will, that there is a life force of divine energy that runs through your body. This life force is known in various circles as the human spirit. We are a unique alchemy of humanity and divinity. Like a river, spirit runs through us with each breath. It is spirit that invigorates the soul. A lack of spirit can literally starve the soul, just as a lack of oxygen can starve each cell. The ways to nurture the soul are countless, yet each ensures a constant flow of this essential life force. Unresolved anger and fear are the two most common ways to choke the human spirit, yet whenever the ego dominates the soul, then the health of the human spirit is diminished. The following are just a few of the many ways to enhance the health of your human spirit. As you read through these ideas, write down, in the form of lists, some ideas of what you can do to engage in these activities, and in doing so engage in the health of your human spirit.

1. **The Art of Self-Renewal:** Self-renewal is a practice of taking time to recharge your personal energy and reconnecting to the divine source of life. List three ways in which you can find time to renew your personal energy—alone. Select the activity, the day and the time of day.

    a._____

    b._____

    c._____

2. **The Practice of Sacred Rituals:** Sacred rituals are traditions that we perform to remind us of the sacredness of life. They include any habit we engage to which we attribute a sense of the divine. List three rituals you partake in on a regular basis to remind you of the sacredness of life.

    a._____

    b._____

    c._____

3. **Embracing the Shadow:** The shadow is a symbol of our dark side, when the ego rules our lives. The shadow appears in the behaviors of prejudice, arrogance, sarcasm, and other less than desirable attributes. To embrace the shadow doesn't mean to exploit these traits, but rather to acknowledge them and work to minimize them. List three aspects of yourself that you find less than flattering. How can you begin to come to peace with these aspects of yourself?

    a._____

    b._____

    c._____

4. **Acts of Forgiveness:** Forgiveness is the antidote for unresolved anger. Every act of forgiveness is an act of unconditional love. When you forgive someone, don't expect an apology. Forgiveness is not the same thing as restitution. Forgiveness is a means of letting go and moving on with your life. A large component of forgiveness is learning to forgive yourself as well. List three people who currently have made it to the top of your "s" list. First write down why you feel violated, and then write down how you can let it go and move on with your life— forgive and start moving freely again.

    a._____

    b._____

    c._____

5. Living Your Joy: First, you cannot live your joy until you can name it. So, name your joy! What things in life give you pleasure, real unconditional happiness, without any sense of regret afterward? Name three things that make you happy and bring a smile to your face. Unresolved stress can inhibit the feelings of joy. List your top three pleasures. When was the last time you did each one of these? How soon can you do them again?

a. _____

b. _____

c. _____

6. Compassion in Action: Compassion in action is pure altruism. It is doing for others without any expectation of reciprocation. Putting compassion into action is putting the work of the soul above the priorities of the ego. Compassion in action begins as random acts of kindness, but it doesn't end there. List three things you can do to express your compassion in action. Is it a random act of kindness? Is it a generous gesture? Or perhaps it is just being there—without feeling a sense of obligation—really being there. Next, set out to do all three of these things on your list.

a. _____

b. _____

c. _____

[CHAPTER 7]

The Keys To Wellness

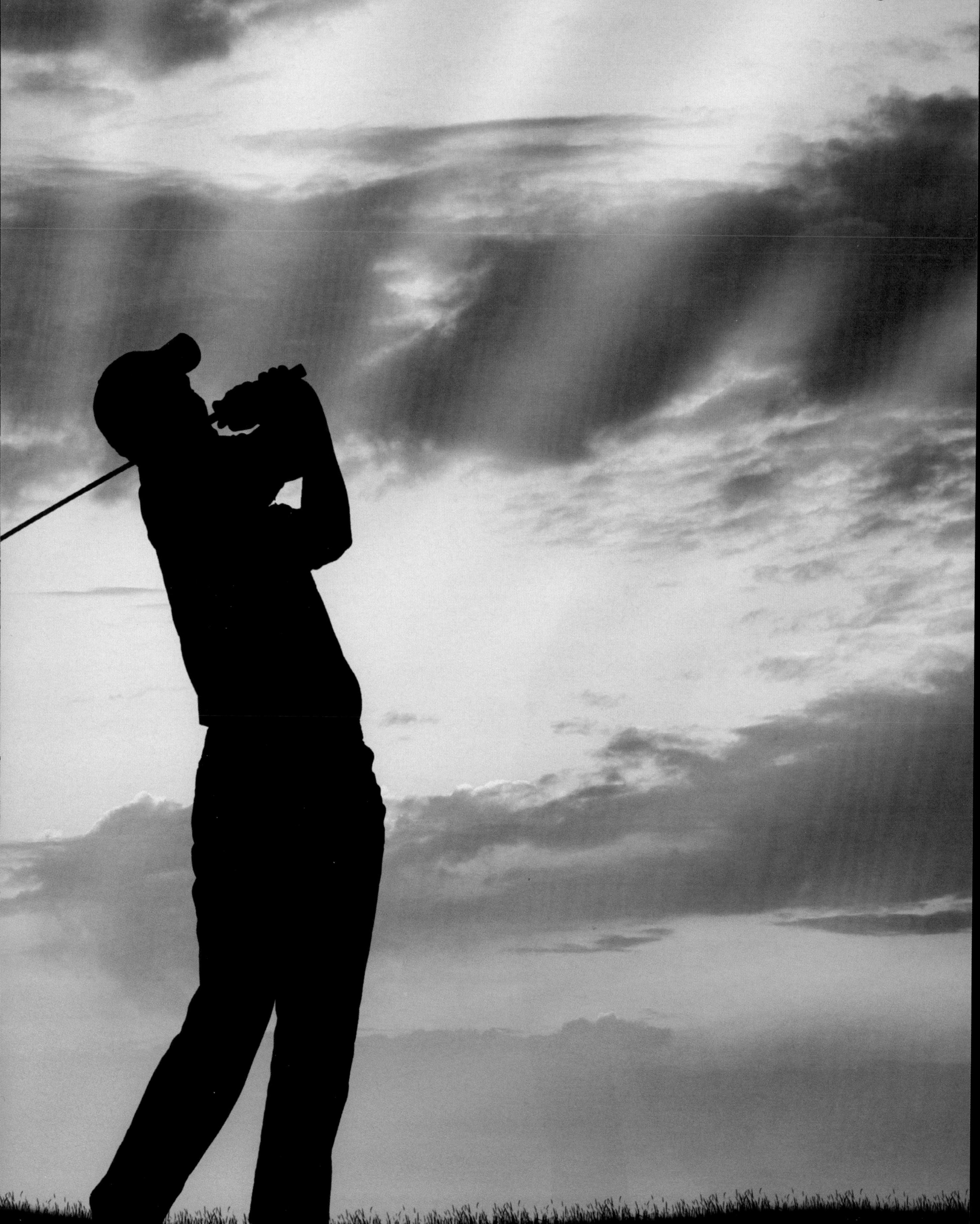

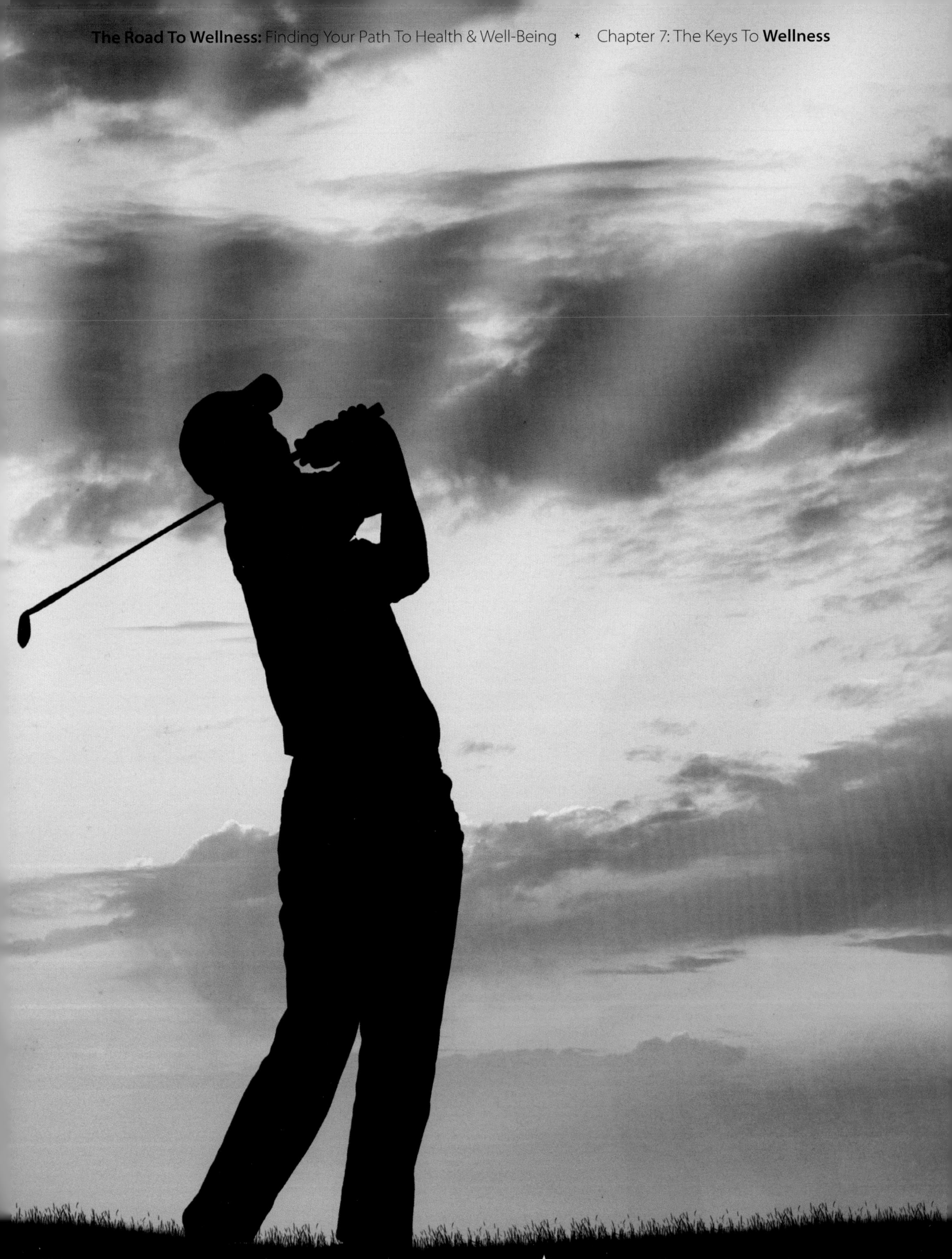

[CHAPTER 7]

The Keys To Wellness

Peter is a young executive who has made it a priority to find a healthy balance between his career and personal life. His motivation? Peter's father dropped dead of a heart attack in a business meeting at age 41. He vowed to live a different lifestyle and he has. He took up surfing and photography at age 30 and the banjo at age 35. Lately, his interests include golf, and in a short time he has become quite good. Over dinner one night Peter said this: "I think playing golf is so much like life in general. Initially, you have to practice the skills to do your best, but ultimately to be good, you can't let it get to your head. I call it finding the 'still point' of pleasure. Outside that still point, you can think so much about your performance that you end up sabotaging your game. This fact applies to life in general." With a smile he added, "I had no idea meditation would be so good for my golf game. I had no idea how good it would be for coping with challenges at work either. There are always things that can throw you off balance, but having a good wellness strategy makes it so much easier to regain your balance. For me, this is the key to life." Peter does not hold a monopoly on this philosophy; it's one we all can and should embrace.

when you have your health, you have everything!

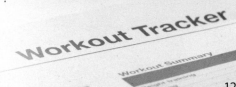

Workout Tracker

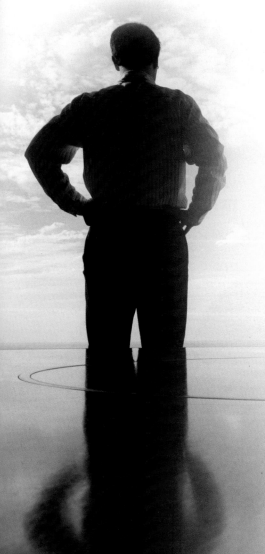

> Here is some sage advice: Skip the rude wake-up call and promise to make your health a daily priority.

Wellness: A Matter Of Priority

As the expression goes, "When you have your health, you have everything!" In our youth, we often take our health for granted. Then, at some point in our 30s (or perhaps even younger) we begin to see that perfect health isn't a guarantee. We have to work at it and never take it for granted. Yet, in a busy world filled with countless responsibilities and distractions, it becomes a bit too easy to forget or ignore good health practices. As a consequence, we let some practical health behaviors slide until we look in the mirror one day and don't recognize the reflection. For some, it takes a rude wake-up call (like a type 2 diabetes diagnosis) to make a radical lifestyle change. For others, like Peter, we are reminded that there is so much more to life than a bank account, a mortgage payment and a fancy car. Health should always be a priority, for without it, the road to the good life can become a tedious, uphill struggle. Taking time each day to eat right, exercise, meditate and laugh are all small investments with both immediate dividends and long-term rewards. Here is some sage advice: Skip the rude wake-up call and promise to make your health a daily priority.

Integration, Balance And Harmony

Our western culture often lives by the motto, "divide and conquer." By separating and reducing things down to a manageable size, it is often easier to comprehend large tasks and undertakings. This same concept has been applied to health and wellness, but not without its consequences. Not seeing the whole picture creates a dangerous blind spot of health. Not only is the topic of health and well-being colossal, but it's also very complex. This, however, we do know; while it may be easy to divide wellness into mental, physical, emotional and spiritual quadrants, there is no separation or division with these components. Our mental health affects our physical health. Our emotions affect our physical health. Our physical health (or lack thereof) can greatly affect our spiritual health. It is all one beautiful, dynamic package. In viewing your health it is essential to see the bigger picture: the integration, balance and harmony of mind, body, spirit and emotions where the whole is always greater than the sum of the parts. This realization is also a key to wellness.

Adaptation

If you have been following the news at all over the past year, you've probably found it hard to overlook the significant global issues that have come knocking on our national (and perhaps personal) door—global warming, economic troubles, rising food prices, water issues, terrorism, etc. While these winds of change (whether they be global or personal) may cause stress, ageless wisdom reminds us that the best way to deal with change is to adapt to it; not fight it and certainly not to ignore it. The same can be said for wellness. The best way to cope with day-to-day life challenges (not to mention the aging process itself) is to adapt with the change. The revered Chinese philosopher Lao Tzu had an expression that bears repeating, "Stand like mountain, flow like water." To stand like a mountain means to be strong, secure and stable in your environment during the winds of change. To flow like water means to let go of the things you cannot control (stop fighting the tide). These are essentially two opposites that when joined together form a bond of wholeness. By no coincidence, this philosophy holds the tenants of successful adaptation. These too are keys to wellness.

Less Is More

As the fire's flames ripped through miles and miles of residential communities along the front range of Colorado from Fort Collins to Colorado Springs, in the summer of 2012 hundreds of people lost their homes, and nearly everything in them that they could not cram in their cars before being forced to evacuate. After the grieving sets in, the realization of starting one's life over begins to take hold. When asked if they would rebuild, many Colorado residents stated that they would move forward with a much smaller house and fewer possessions; they would have less, not more things. This is good advice for all of us.

If you were to study the lifestyles of people living a few generations ago you would see that, by and large, people lived within their means. This fact was really put to the test during the Great Depression and once again during World War II. People can become quite creative in order to make ends meet and enjoy the simple pleasures of life. In our current age of the entitlement generation, things are quite different. We live in a culture of abundance (particularly when compared to other global communities) yet too much of a good thing (e.g., comfort foods, technology, etc.) is not good at all. The ability to "have it all" is coming back to haunt us. Once again, freedom to choose must be balanced with the responsibility to act.

It has been said that Americans have become complacent. Although there may be several reasons this is often a consequence of enjoying the good life a little too much. Balance is key! As these global events and national headlines remind us, the winds of change are in the air. How can we learn to scale back…and still be happy? The answer is this: less is more. In the words of the renowned sailor Robin Lee Graham who circumnavigated the world alone at age 16: "It's not how much you need to get by, it's how little you need to get by."

> "Once again, freedom to choose must be balanced with the responsibility to act."

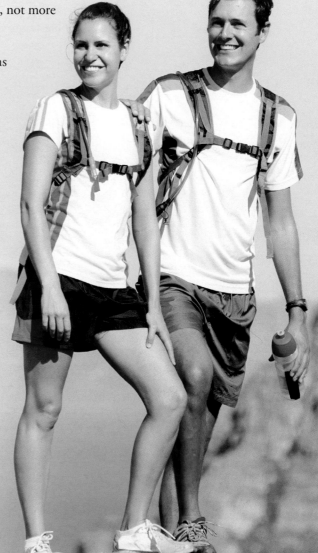

> The keys to the good life include a healthy attitude, persistance, perspiration, inspiration, a good sense of humor, resiliency and an open heart.

Wellness: The Next Step

The good life is often symbolized as a photo of two successful young people sipping a cool umbrella drink under the shade of a palm tree on a secluded island beach. While this certainly symbolizes a good life moment, the real good life is a multitude of moments, alone or together with friends, where at any point throughout your lifespan you can sit and appreciate all of your life experiences with few, if any, regrets. The keys to the good life include a healthy attitude, persistence, perspiration, inspiration, a good sense of humor, resiliency and an open heart. The good news is that these keys are in your hands right now.

Reading this book and completing the worksheets, questionnaires and surveys constitutes the first step in establishing and maintaining your personal wellness program, but there is no substitute for personal experience. Putting your wellness program into action takes action. To repeat the expression, "To know and not to do is not to know." It's time to "do." Your next step toward the good life awaits you.

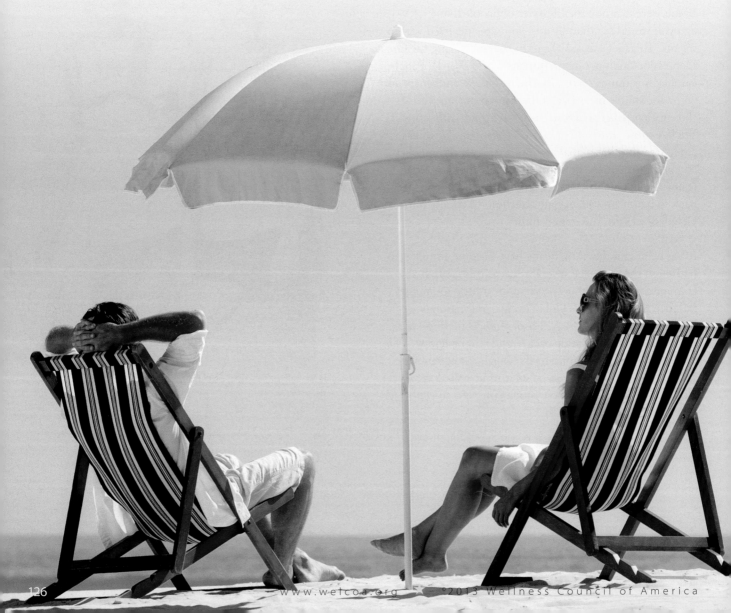